What others are say.

"For those who are interested in making positive changes in all aspects of their lives, *Healthspan* is the book to read. Jack and Genevieve Woodard spell out in clear detail the means of achieving a peaceful mind, a joyful spirit, and an energetic, well-functioning body. This information they present is precise, solidly scientific, and full of a wholesome philosophy of life that will fill you with a sense of urgency to begin applying their techniques immediately. This is a landmark book that can not only add years to your life, but will markedly improve your mental and physical health during those extra years."

—A. Vernon Dixon, M.D., Child and Adolescent Psychiatrist

"Having been through death's door and back again, not only to the land of the living, but to robust health, I owe my life to Jack Woodard. Yes, I know healing really comes from God, but He certainly used Jack as His instrument. Here, in *Healthspan,* are powerful, dynamic, life changing strategies to benefit everyone on this planet. This book is a must read!"

—Melba Corbett-Moreth, N.D.

"The healthcare system of the future is predicated on people taking greater responsibility for their own health. *Healthspan* is essential for those who wish to do so. This book is an indispensable resource that can help you and your family protect your health, live with vitality, and enhance your body's natural healing ability. It is vital to those who seriously desire to reduce their risk of chronic disease and improve their quality of life. An excellent and much needed resource. Motivating and inspiring."

— J. Michael Dierkes, DDS, MS, FICCMO, Former Director,
Peachtree Health and Wellness Associates

Healthspan

Claim Your Birthright to Holistic Health and Happiness from Here to 100

O. Jack Woodard, Jr., M.D
Genevieve Johnson Woodard

Healthspirit Press, Clayton, Georgia

Healthspan
Claim your Birthright to Holistic Health
and Happiness from Here to 100
Copyright © 2000 by O. Jack Woodard, Jr., M.D.

Published by: ☙ Healthspirit Press
Post Office Box 806
Clayton, GA 30525-0806 U.S.A.

Publisher's Cataloging-in-Publication
(Provided by Quality Books, Inc.)
Woodard, O. Jack
    Healthspan : claim your birthright to holistic
    health and happiness from here to 100 / O. Jack
    Woodard, Genevieve Johnson-Woodard. -- 1st ed.
    p. cm.
    Includes bibliographical references and index.
    LCCN: 99-95248
    ISBN: 0-9671247-0-0

    1. Longevity. 2. Self-care, Health
I. Johnson-Woodard, Genevieve. II. Title.

RA776.75.W66 1999   612.6'8
                    QB199-945

10 9 8 7 6 5 4 3 2 1

PRINTED IN THE UNITED STATES OF AMERICA

Dedication

To Andrew Ralston Woodard
24 September 1964 - 23 September 1985
for the joy and laughter he brought into our
lives and for teaching us so much
about living and dying.

The path of the just is as the shining light that shineth more and more unto the perfect day.

—Proverbs 4:18

TABLE OF CONTENTS

Appendix

Foreword

Most of us want to live longer, and stay healthy while growing older. Those of us reading this book have probably been attracted by the promise of its title, and are not surprised after scanning the contents pages that the approach appears to be through holistic health practices. So, what's new and special about that?

"Holistic" health has been a major theme in books, magazines, and other media for over a decade. We're urged to eat right and eat less, exercise more, take our vitamins, minerals and herbs, meditate, pray, do acupuncture, massage, and chiropractic...the list goes on and on. When applied by physicians and other practitioners, these individual approaches are frequently mislabeled "holistic medicine". In reality, "holistic medicine" is infrequently practiced. Originally (and more accurately) spelled "wholistic", the name refers to the "whole picture" of health: physical, mental, and spiritual.

Medical practitioners who actually are "holistic" in their approach are harder to find than one might think. Most of us specialize in one or more of the 'parts of the whole' noted above. Patients and friends of Dr. Jack Woodard and Genevieve Woodard are especially fortunate to have available to them *real* holistic medicine, in the original and best sense of the term.

That's what makes this book special among books about achieving good health. It not only explains, blends and intertwines the physical, mental, and spiritual aspects of holistic health, showing how each part affects the others, but it goes beyond that, asking (and even more importantly, *answering*) the obvious but usually-neglected question: "What is good health *for*?"

If we don't know the answer to this question, then we're not as likely to achieve the good health we're looking for. Like the dog forever chasing the car, we won't know what to do with it if we ever do catch it! As Dr. Freud (who is correct occasionally) would have told us, the subconscious mind knows if we've truly answered "what is good health *for*?", and if we haven't, it may not help us or even hinder us on the road to the good health the conscious mind desires.

If there's no *reason* to live to 100 years or more, we probably won't! Diet, physical conditioning, meditation, and all of the multiple aspects of holistic health are literally "empty exercises" without a purpose. If the Woodards had made only that point in what follows, it would be worthwhile. But like true holistic practitioners, they include much more, and give us valuable tools, insights, and advice about achieving the best physical, mental, and spiritual health we can, so we can best **use** our good health for the reasons and purposes unique to each one of us.

—Jonathan V. Wright, M.D.

Preface

This book is both professional and personal. Some of it is an account of the most important things we lave learned during many years of clinical work and teaching. Some of it chronicles our struggles, successes, and failures in our search for an ideal way of life. We have used our stories and those of our families for illustrations — not because our stories are better or more interesting, but because we know our families and ourselves better than we know any other. On the professional level, *Healthspan* is the distillation of the knowledge Jack has gained in over 40 years of medical practice and what I have gained in working as his co-therapist and co-worker for over 25 years.

One of the attributes that makes Jack a great physician is his insatiable thirst for knowledge. He is always looking for better ways to treat his patients, as well as ways to find more health and peace in his own life. This is great for his medical practice, but it surely is a disadvantage in getting a book to a publisher! We finally had to agree that this book would be about what he has learned to a certain point; anything new he learns after that day goes into the next book.

Originally my thinking was that Jack would author the entire book; I would proof and make suggestions. As the book went through many transformations over a period of three years, I became more involved in the actual writing of the manuscript. Although we have each contributed to every chapter in some way, Jack has contributed the medical and scientific aspects. I have written, "Strengthening the Power of Attention" and "Relationships". Except for those two chapters where "I" belongs to me, the other chapters are primarily Jack's work. The "I" in those chapters belongs to him. Many times we have agreed on the concepts and have used "we".

For about ten years, we knew a couple whom we will call Joe and Jane. During that time, many different things happened to their family and to ours, some quite painful. In their family, the first major stress was Joe's retirement. Later, their only child went through heartbreaking divorce. Another painful thing was the illness and death of Jane's mother, who was in her nineties and had been an invalid. In the few months following these two severe stresses, Jane became almost nonfunctional. She sat in her living room with a shawl around her shoulders for hours. Joe did all of the cooking, bought the groceries, and did the house cleaning. He did all of the work that she had been doing while she just sat in the chair. When I asked her how she was doing, she would say, "I'm just under so much stress."

During those same years, our younger son Andy died the night before his twenty-first birthday; and a few years later during the great flood of 1994, we lost many personal possessions as well as most of our office equipment and records. We had left all of our family portraits at the office in storage while we built our house and just never did move them to the house. Our daughter's wedding dress, antiques from the Woodard family and many other personal mementos went down in the flood. The only thing left usable as far as the office itself was concerned was the 2 x 4's throughout the building, the cypress wood exterior, the roof and the front porch. Everything else had to be gutted.

When we were finally allowed to enter our office two weeks after the flood, my first thought as I viewed the unbelievable devastation was that what we had lost was primarily material things that we could replace if we made enough money. The pictures and other personal effects were well enough etched in my memory that I could do without them.

Jack's remark as he coped with our loss from the flood was that what made him a physician is in his head, his heart, and his hands. The loss of the building and its contents did not diminish his ability to continue fulfilling his purpose in life. Neither Jack nor I shed a tear over losing the office, although it put us under heavy financial stress that continues to this day. At the rate we are going, we will be out of debt when we are 79 years old!

Nothing that had happened in my life up to that point prepared me for the searing pain, agony, and grief that I experienced after Andy died. I had the belief that, if I were a good mother, I would protect my children. The most helpless feeling I have had by far was watching our beloved son suffer and die and not being able to do a thing about it. For several weeks after Andy's death I stayed close to home and experienced my grief to its fullest. At night when I could not sleep, I kicked myself unmercifully for not having been a better mother to him. I did not go out and do my normal activities except for walking, because I never knew when I would get a flashback to his last days with us and start crying. Waves of grief would flow over me at times that seemed to be so severe that I feared that I could not cope with it. Then for a while my mood would brighten and I could again count my blessings. However, I didn't have control over what would come when!

About six weeks after Andy died, I realized that I was still alive and I had not completed the mission that God put me on this earth to do. It was time for me to get up and get busy fulfilling my purpose again. I regained my functioning to the place that I was able to go back to work and to resume my playing the piano and organ for church and entertaining friends. The pain over losing the physical presence of our son did not go away and probably never will; it lessens in severity each time we are able to use what we learned from his illness and death in assisting our fellow travelers cope with their heartbreaks and losses. Finally, after nearly 14 years, when I think of Andy I breathe a prayer of thanksgiving that I was allowed to have his physical presence for 21 years. I am grateful for all the things he taught me.

What made the difference in the way the two families responded to crises during these years? I cannot say for sure because I have never walked in their shoes. However, I do know that in the late 1960's Jack and I began putting together a stress management program that has really worked for us. In the late 1960's, we started jogging three miles six days a week. We found that we could continue our exercise in South Georgia just about every day of the year if we could just get out early enough on hot summer mornings.

The next step in our managing stress occurred in the early 1970's when we began studying Bowen's Family Systems Theory at Georgetown University. Here we learned, among many other very useful things that you will read about in the chapter on relationships, how to develop a support system, and how to bring down the level of stress at home.

In the mid 1970's we began meditating. Jack learned more about nutrition; we began to clean up our diet and our style of living. Our children were teenagers at this point, so I phased in healthful, nutritious food very gradually.

Probably one of the most important things we did with our stress management program was to become fully aware of what our purpose is in being on this earth, not only as individuals but also as a family. Once we became clear on what our mission in life is, we were able to set our priorities much better. We began to leave off things that did not help us fulfill our mission, so when the big stresses and heartaches came into our lives, we had a good stress management program in place.

What I would like to add to Jack's introduction is that *this system works*! I am reminded of the saying, "It isn't the weight of the load that gets you down; it is how you carry it."

Yes, we have had our stressful times and our heartaches, and we have shed many tears; but we have always known that weeping would be just for the night and joy would come in the morning.

—Genevieve Johnson Woodard

Introduction

Since I was a boy, I have known that it is my mission is to participate in the process of solving the problem of suffering. When I was in middle school, I took a first aid kit out on the playground during recess so I could dress my schoolmates' inevitable cuts and scrapes. There was usually plenty of business, but I eventually realized that Band Aids and antiseptic were not going to be enough to solve the problem of suffering. During those years, I lay awake at night for hours, spinning elaborate fantasies about curing people's diseases and sharing their happiness as they returned to health.

During adolescence, my attention turned to darker, more hormonally driven matters. Then, when I was 17, I had a conversion experience at a church retreat. With it, the awareness of mission returned just in time for me to enter a premedical curriculum in college. During the college years, it seemed to me that the solution to the problem of suffering was in the mind. That was certainly where most of mine was happening. I was drawn to the study of psychology.

In medical school, I gravitated toward psychiatry and found that I had an aptitude for it. After graduation, I entered a psychiatric residency, completed it, and began private practice.

The first few, frustrating years in practice taught me that psychiatry, while more effective than Band Aids and Merthiolate, was a three-foot leap across a six-foot ditch when it came to solving the problem of suffering. I had to acknowledge that mind and body are inextricably interconnected and that the suffering of each has to be addressed if the problem is to be solved. That sobering discovery motivated me to add the physical interventions of diet and exercise. The idea that such things could have anything to do with health and happiness was so preposterous to most people in the '60's, that it was a hard sell. The few patients who followed the new prescription did attain more reduction in their suffering than the rest.

The biggest breakthrough came in 1975, when, driven by my own intense mental suffering, I began to meditate. This had such a salutary effect on my suffering and health that I had to prescribe it for my patients. It worked so well for most of the ones who did it that it has been an important part of my holistic prescription ever since.

By that time, I finally had a holistic program, addressing the physical, mental, and spiritual levels of life, to offer for the relief of suffering. It was not perfect and it did not work as well as I wished, but it was far better than anything I had used before. I used it happily for a decade until another crisis blew my world apart and set me searching again.

In the mid '80's, a death in my family showed me that all I had assembled to help people was still inadequate. In response to this agonizing lesson, I studied orthomolecular medicine and got training in environmental and ayurvedic medicine. Ayurveda gave me the framework upon which I could organize the best of all I had learned into a truly holistic therapeutic system.

With developments and discoveries in holistic medicine coming at a constantly accelerating rate, the therapeutic system is constantly evolving. As it does so, it becomes more effective for the fulfillment of my mission to participate in the solution to the problem of suffering.

What *Healthspan* is about

Life is not living, but living in health.

—Marcus Valarius Martialis

Healthspan is about claiming or losing a fabulously rich birthright. It is also about the three most important discoveries that we have gained from our combined 66 years of clinical practice and teaching and our 130 years on earth. The discoveries are about living in health and happiness for a long time. They are:

- We are rightful heirs to the birthright of the 100-year healthspan: living with zest, vigor, fulfillment, physical, mental, and spiritual well-being—and a predominance of comfort over discomfort until the age of 100 years or more.

- Powerful forces will, if we do not counteract them, deny our access to claiming and enjoying our birthright. These forces include environmental pollution, a degraded food supply, dangerous mutations in bacteria and viruses, abusive lifestyles, superstition, and ignorance. Each of these acts on one or more of the three most important levels of life: physical, mental, and spiritual.

- There are effective countermeasures to neutralize each of these negative forces. Since the negative forces affect all three levels of life, the appropriate countermeasures must be applied on each level. You can learn to use these countermeasures effectively and make them fun, fascinating, and feasible in real life and in real time. This is how you conquer the negative forces and claim your birthright.

Who should read this book?

People who:

- believe there is more to life and health than they are experiencing

- feel confused and overwhelmed by the flood of information and conflicting health claims filling the media

- are uninsured and afraid of financial and physical disaster if they get sick

- know that the magic bullet approach of conventional medicine is often inadequate and sometimes produces painful or deadly ricochets

- want a practical, clinically proven, holistic program, developed by a medical doctor over a period of more than 40 years, for achieving maximum health

- are intrigued by the idea that Nature intends human beings to be healthy and happy for 100 years or more, and want to see some evidence for it

- wish to use natural interventions to enhance benefit from conventional medical treatment. This is especially important for those who have life threatening, disabling, or chronic diseases for which conventional medicine has no cure and can only suppress symptoms.

- already know, or almost know, some of what they will read in this book, but are afraid to act on it because they don't know anyone else, particularly any experienced M.D., who knows it.

Why you should read Healthspan

I saw a highway of diamonds with nobody on it.

—Bob Dylan

1. **For evidence that it is possible.** One of the main dangers to claiming your birthright is that you do not believe that it exists. After all, you may never have seen, or even heard of, anyone who enjoyed health and happiness until the age of a hundred or more. What you have never seen or heard about, you may consider impossible. What you consider impossible, you probably won't bother to learn about, much less attempt. Therefore, the first chapter of the book presents some of the evidence that the 100-year healthspan is possible—not only possible, but Nature's precious birthright to human beings.

2. **For knowledge of the hazards.** If the evidence convinces you that the 100-year healthspan may be possible, or if you already know that it is, you may want to know why you don't see many people achieving it. In the second chapter, "Dream Destroyers and Birthright Burglars," we describe what we have learned about the five most dangerous things that keep people from attaining the 100-year healthspan. There are some pretty scary, heavy things in this section—some bad news. However, there is good news about the bad news. The good news is that for

every hazard and danger there are effective countermeasures. You'll find out about them in Section II, "Knowledge for Claiming Your Birthright." I thought about calling the second section "Defusing Dream Destroyers and Bashing Birthright Burglars," but it's much more than that. It focuses on things that are proactive, powerful, interesting, and enjoyable—things that lead out of suffering into fulfillment, health, and happiness.

3. **For different strokes for different folks.** This is the only book I know written by two soul mates who are in the forty-fifth year of their marriage. Genevieve and I are living proof that opposites attract. We both are strong, independent, opinionated, articulate, determined people, who have differing views on many important subjects. Finding unity in such diversity has been a powerful, ongoing learning experience that continues to this day. In more than four decades of living intimately together, we have walked through heaven and hell barefooted—several times. These experiences have taught us much about how to solve the problem of suffering. Since we are so different, we bring to this book a range of perspective that it would be impossible for one author to achieve. This makes the knowledge in this book uniquely able to address the needs and situations of an extraordinarily wide range of individuals. Our differing styles and approaches are complementary and provide a richness of communication and content that many readers are likely to find enjoyable and helpful.

4. **For passion and seasoned judgment.**
Go with passion, but go with skillful, seasoned passion.

— OJW

Another unusual feature of this book is that I have grown up with the renaissance of holistic medicine. For many years, I have watched the evolution of this field, participated in it, and have seen many health fads come and go. This has given me a seasoned, practical judgment about what works and what does not. This can be valuable to people who are just becoming acquainted with the field of holistic medicine and natural therapies and feel bewildered by the explosion of information, misinformation, and disinformation that is filling the media. From a vast array of things you *might* do to improve health, I present the six that, in my experience, are the most powerful for most people. This reduces a bewildering diversity to an exciting and entirely feasible starting point for a magnificent adventure.

I am passionate about the practice of holistic medicine and about the teaching of holistic health skills. After all, medical practice and teaching are major ways of fulfilling my life mission to participate in the solution to the problem of suffering. This passion is balanced by over 40 years of clinical experience. The balance provides both of us some protection against my practicing and teaching with more enthusiasm than skill.

5. **For balance and harmony.** Another feature that sets this book apart from hundreds of other self help books is that it appreciates and teaches the necessity of creating balance and harmony on the three most important levels of life: spiritual, mental, and physical. The Healthspan System works on all these levels and works on them simultaneously. This is essential to success in the quest for the 100-year healthspan because, contrary to the fond hope of most people, there is no magic bullet that will do the job. From time to time, someone thinks he has discovered the magic bullet but eventually, alas, it ricochets or falls short of the mark.

6. **For knowledge** (which is power) and wisdom (which is superpower). Knowledge tells you how to achieve balance on each of the three levels of life. Wisdom is necessary to get and keep all three levels of life balanced with each other. In Chapter 13: "Balancing Whole Self, Strategy," we tell you how to cultivate this wisdom. This technology for the development of wisdom is one of the most valuable contributions of *Healthspan*

What is in it

This book is divided into three sections:

Section 1: The Possible Dream describes our discovery of our birthright, presents our evidence for the feasibility of the 100-year healthspan, and the hazards against it.

Section 2: Knowledge for Claiming Your Birthright tells you things you can do on the spiritual, mental, and physical levels of life to defeat the dream destroyers, baffle the birthright burglars and win the 100-year healthspan in spite of them. The power of attention is the master key, so we devote three chapters to telling you what it is, how to apply it, and how to get more of it. On the mental level, we describe how to master the ego, discover and fulfill your life mission, and cultivate relationships that are more fulfilling than frustrating. On the physical plane, we give you the technology for building and balancing your life energy, or *chi*, and using food and nutritional supplements to balance and optimize your biochemistry. Here you will learn about some exciting and powerful new breakthroughs.

Section 3: Wisdom for Claiming Your Birthright teaches you the process of tapping your deep inner wisdom to integrate what you learned in the first two sections into a personalized program that is right for you in your real world circumstances now—and will not only work, but be fun, fascinating, and user friendly. There is a chapter on creating your unique strategy for attaining your 100-year healthspan. The final chapter suggests winning tactics for successfully carrying out your strategy. It gives systematic suggestions about how to get started.

How to use this book

There are at least three options:

1. Read it through from start to finish.

2. If you wish to begin the Healthspan Program before you finish the book, read Chapter 14: *Tactics*. You will find implementation instructions there. They will refer you to the parts of Section 2 and the Appendix where you learn how to do the interventions you have selected. There are two advantages to exercising this option: you begin to enjoy the adventure and its benefits sooner and, as you concurrently do the program and continue to read about it,

you learn why the system works and the mechanics by which you are creating the benefits you are appreciating.

3. If you are not interested in the metaphysics of the 100-year healthspan, but just want to experience it as soon as possible, skim or skip the parts of Chapters 5, 6, and 7 that deal with the Whole Self. For that matter, skim or skip any parts of Section 2 that do not interest you now. You may wish to read those parts later. The book is so content-rich that you will need to read it more than once to get maximum benefit. The metaphysics will be more interesting in a subsequent reading, after you have felt the healing power of the procedures they explain.

—O. Jack Woodard, Jr., M.D.

ACKNOWLEDGEMENTS

In the 1980's, our seminar students began asking for a book containing the information that we were teaching. We always provided an extensive bibliography, but much of the material we were teaching was from our own experiences. We were on such a steep learning curve that we knew that it was not time to put the information into a book but we are grateful to those students and patients who repeatedly encouraged us to "Put it into print." They planted the seed and kept before us the idea of writing a book.

We are deeply indebted to our children, Marian Lee Woodard, and Jack Woodard III, for their encouragement, love, and support and for supplying us with the equipment we needed, including two computers and a printer. Without these, it is unlikely that we would have completed this book. Our son-in-law, John Matthesen, gave us valuable technical support as we learned to use the computers.

Genevieve's brother, Andrew Myron Johnson, M.D., gave unstintingly of his time and extensive scientific and editorial expertise. He read the entire manuscript and suggested many improvements. His thorough editing made the book stronger and more readable.

We are indebted to Bart Flick, M.D., for the Flick Protocol that is featured in the book. He and his wife, Bonnie, gave us much needed encouragement, emotional support, and suggestions.

Deepak Chopra, M.D. widened and deepened the world of holistic medicine for us with his *Quantum Healing*. His many subsequent books and tapes have nurtured us in the process of integrating ayurveda with modern science and medicine. His insights and wisdom have enriched our lives, this book and our abilities to serve our patients and students. He has permitted us to quote him in this volume. We are deeply indebted to him.

Sidney M. Baker, M.D. has taught me most of what I know about the process of practicing holistic medicine. He is a master teacher, spicing vital information with a scintillating humor. His Tacks

Laws, sprinkled throughout this book are examples. I will always be grateful to him for making it fun to gain such valuable knowledge.

Dr. Wayne Dyer, with his book and audiotape album, *Real Magic,* showed us how to present information about the power of consciousness to people unfamiliar with the metaphysical. I have prescribed *Real Magic* to many patients. The effect has been magical for those who took the prescription. I have written about some of these in *Healthspan.* Dr. Dyer continues to inspire us, most recently with *Manifest Your Destiny.* We particularly appreciate his quote on page 200.

Jeffrey Bland, Ph.D., president and CEO of HealthCom International, Inc. and editor of *Functional Medicine Update,* has been an unfailing source of timely, and ahead of timely, information about the biochemical aspects of holistic medical practice. He is usually at least a decade ahead of the curve. After I hear about something from Jeff, I often see it 10 or 15 years later in the *New England Journal of Medicine* or the AMA Journal. We appreciate his permission to use an inspiring story about his grandfather in the Epilogue.

Dr. Stephen Covey has enhanced the quality of life of our whole family and many of our patients and students with his *The 7 Habits of Highly Effective People.* His system works. His dry wit makes learning enjoyable. The quote on page 52 is memorable. His protocol for discovering life mission, described in Chapter 8, is among the best.

James Redfield is a prime mover in the global expansion of consciousness now ongoing. His writings have certainly expanded ours—andat crucial times. His insights have added value to this book and have been a blessing to our patients and students. His quote on page 94 is a good example of his power to convey profound truth concisely.

Caroline Myss, Ph.D., in *Enery Anatomy,* gave us a practical, powerful way to apply energy medicine. Our patients and we are benefiting from her insight and wisdom.

Denny Ray Johnson generously allowed us to publish his startingly effective protocol for clearing negative energy from the family tree. It adds a unique dimension to energy healing. He has made a significant contribution to the value of this book.

Alston Griffin has done more than our graphic design. She has understood and appreciated the spirit of *Healthspan,* guided us in the book production process, been available on weekends to accommodate our unusual clinical schedule in Atlanta, and has energized and encouraged us.

Many of our patients, students, and friends read parts or all of the manuscript and made helpful suggestions. Among them are Amy Villarreal, Peggy Groves, Melba Corbett-Moreth, N.D., J. Michael Dierkes, DDS, Bernola Paschal, RN., and Bill and Miriam Foster.

We would like to thank our patients who wrote about their experiences with holistic medicine and permitted us to share them with you.

The four lines quoted on page 86 are from *Poems of Sidney Lanier,* copyright 1944, edited by his wife.

The seven lines quoted in the first paragraph on page 93 are from *The Dhammapada,* copyright 1976 by Thomas Byrom, translated by Thomas Byrom.

The seven lines quoted on page 138 are from *The Healing Path of Prayer,* copyright 1997 by Ron Roth and Peter Occhiogrosso, by Ron Roth and Peter Occhiogrosso.

The lines quoted on pages 20 and 234 are from *Writings and Drawings by Bob Dylan,* copyright 1973 by Bob Dylan, by Bob Dylan.

The two lines on page 235 are from *The Prophet,* copyright 1951 by Mary Gibran, by Kahlil Gibran.

The last two lines on page 348 are from *Gitanjali,* copyright 1971 by Macmillan Publishing Co., by Rabindranath Tagore.

To all the above, and to the many others who gave us suggestions and encouragement at crucial times, we owe a debt of gratitude. Thank you!

The heart has arguments with which the logic of the mind is not acquainted.

—Blaise Paschal

Warning-Disclaimer

This book is designed to provide information about ways and means of attaining the highest probability of enjoying the 100-year healthspan. It is sold with the understanding that the authors are not prescribing medical treatment without first examining the patient. This information is intended to complement the advice of your personal physician, not replace it.

It is not the purpose of this book to reprint all of the information that is otherwise available to the authors, but to complement, amplify, and supplement other texts. You are urged to read all of the available material, learn as much as possible about the attainment of your 100-year healthspan, and to tailor the information to your individual needs. For more information, see the many references throughout the text.

Every effort has been made to make this book as complete and as accurate as possible. However, **there may be typographical or content mistakes.** Therefore, this text should be used only as a general guide and not as the ultimate source of health enhancement information. Furthermore, this book contains information on health enhancement only up to the printing date.

The purpose of this book is to educate and entertain. The authors and Healthspirit Press shall have neither liability nor responsibility to any person or entity with respect to loss or damage caused, or alleged to be caused, directly or indirectly by the information contained in this book.

If you do not wish to be bound by the above, you may return this book to the publisher for a full refund.

About the Authors

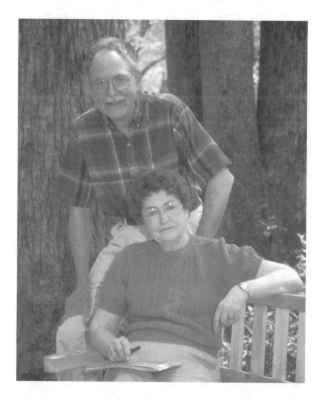

Jack Woodard has known since childhood that his life mission is to participate in solving the problem of suffering. To prepare himself, he went to medical school and completed a psychiatric residency. He soon learned that these skills, while valuable, were insufficient. He continued his quest for more adequate means for mission fulfillment. The path led through nutritional medicine, environmental medicine, Zen, ayurvedic medicine, and energy medicine. As he traversed each field, he brought with him the procedures and technology that worked best for his patients, eventually integrating them all into the unique, holistic system that is the subject of this book.

Dr. Woodard is Board certified in psychiatry. He has served as Chief of Staff and as Chief of Psychiatry at Phoebe Putney Memorial Hospital in Albany, Georgia. Since 1995, he has practiced holistic medicine in Clayton, Georgia, and in Atlanta. He lectures on applications of holistic medicine and appears on talk shows. With Genevieve Johnson-Woodard, he founded Healthspan Center for the practice of holistic medicine and for holistic education. Together, they lead workshops on different aspects of holistic health enhancement for the attainment of the 100-year healthspan.

His hobbies include organic gardening, hiking, and cutting firewood for warmth during the mountain winters.

Genevieve Johnson-Woodard is a teacher by talent and training. After honing her skills in public school classrooms, she began, in the 1970's, to teach health enhancement and relationship skills. She has post graduate training in Transactional Analysis and in Family Systems Therapy.

She lectures on living skills, stress management, cultivation of high quality relationships, and the holistic approach to the 100-year healthspan. Her style combines warmth, wit, and wisdom in a way that can move her audiences alternately to laughter and to tears.

Her teaching includes individual instruction to patients on how to do the holistic procedures that Dr. Woodard prescribes for them. She and Dr. Woodard serve as co-therapists for families and individuals with complex and difficult problems.

She is a talented musician, playing piano and organ for churches and musical groups. Her hobbies include gardening, gourmet cooking, hiking, and travel.

Jack and Genevieve have two children, now adults, who are fulfilling their own life missions in ways that make their parents happy and proud.

Believe that life is worth living and your belief will create the fact.

—William James

Part I
The Possible Dream:
Your 100-Year
Healthspan

Chapter 1

DEATH, DELIVERANCE, and DISCOVERY

The death was our son's. The deliverance was our patients'—and our own. The discovery was a fabulous birthright from Nature. **Healthspan** *is the story of how they are connected—and what it can mean to you.*

Deliverance

"Ken, your liver tests are completely normal!"

My voice sounded strange, affected by a combination of excitement, joy, and awe. I looked into his eyes to see if he understood what the normal liver tests meant. He understood. I felt my own eyes sting with tears of gratitude and happiness.

I was sitting in my consulting room with Ken, a 68-year-old dentist who was under a death sentence because of advanced liver cancer. The cancer had become so extensive that his oncologist would not give him chemotherapy. His daughter, who had achieved powerful healing through a recovery program she and I worked out together, had said to Ken, "For God's sake, Daddy, go see Jack Woodard. I believe he can help you."

Ken and I had developed a holistic recovery program that included a vegetarian diet, comprehensive nutritional support with large doses of co-enzyme Q-10, as much vitamin C as he could swallow without getting diarrhea, and two or three infusions per week of vitamin C 20 grams (20,000 milligrams), B vitamins, and magnesium. From Genevieve, he had learned how to meditate and use visual imagery to strengthen his immune system. He was walking daily in a beautiful mountain forest near his home. He spent plenty of time sitting on a rock in the woods, absorbed in the beauty and healing power of nature. He cultivated a friendship network at a church where he felt love and inspiration. Over the past months his strength and experience of well being had increased until he was enjoying better quality of life than he had before he got cancer. People were telling him that he looked healthier than he had in years.

We were regularly doing blood tests for his liver enzymes and bilirubin, which had been very high while cancer was destroying his liver. We had seen the enzyme and bilirubin levels fall toward normal with each successive test. That day, I had been so excited that I could hardly wait for Ken to arrive. The current battery of liver tests showed normal function! Ken and I sat together, looking at those wonderful numbers on his lab report and thanked God from the depths of our hearts. Ken said, "My oncologist told me I would be dead before the first of this year. Now I've seen the leaves come out on the trees this spring."

I said, "Yes, and if you can avoid getting run over by a truck, you will probably see them turn red this fall, too."

Ken phoned a few weeks ago to let us know that, after two years, there is still no sign of cancer. He believes that had it not been for the work we did together, he would be dead. He encouraged me to use his real name in this book and offered to talk to anyone who wished to know more about his healing.

Life and health are about balance and harmony. Ken used these principles to create a medical miracle out of a death sentence. My participation in the grace and joy of Ken's deliverance helped me balance the most devastating experience of my life, 11 years earlier.

Death

Andy was dying. For a week, he had lain on an airbed in an intensive care unit of a teaching hospital of a major medical school. His usually lean, lithe 20-year-old body and handsome face were grotesquely bloated and his skin was in shreds from a violent allergic reaction to antibiotics that were supposed to treat pneumonia. He was attached to life support systems by various tubes, wires, and a respirator hose. His bone marrow had been destroyed by one too many rounds of chemotherapy for Hodgkin's Disease. Unable to make white blood cells, his body was helpless against the onslaught of *Pneumocystis* bacteria and *Candida* yeast. The intravenous antibiotics and fungicides were poisoning him faster than they were killing the organisms that were killing him.

He had slipped into a coma several hours earlier. Genevieve, his sister, brother, fiancée, and I had watched the numbers on his blood pressure monitor slip below the level that was compatible with life. We saw his EKG tracing change to a pattern that a nurse said was terminal. His fiancée, who had been by his side throughout most of the past week, was holding his left hand. His brother and sister were standing at the foot of the bed each touching one of Andy's feet. With my hand on Andy's right shoulder, I was softly chanting into his ear a Zen verse for serenity, reassurance, and enlightenment. His mother was sitting a few feet away with a group of the closest friends of the family. They were sending to Andy a current of love that flowed through the suffocating hospital atmosphere like a cool mountain breeze across a parched desert.

Two hundred miles to the south, Andy's Sheltie was howling continuously beside the door through which Andy had left the house for the last time. The sun set. The last light faded on the day of the autumnal equinox. The blood pressure monitor showed zeros. The EKG tracing went flat, except for an artifact in the instrument. Andy's spirit slipped free of his body which had been damaged beyond repair. It was four hours before his twenty-first birthday. Andy was our youngest child.

In the desolation and suffocating grief following his death, I had formed an implacable resolve to do whatever I could do to spare anyone else what Andy suffered and what his mother, brother, sister, fiancée, and I experienced. This drove me into a quest for new knowledge that led to some strange and unexpected places and experiences. I expanded the study of nutritional medicine that I had begun when I learned, two years before his death, that Andy had cancer. The study of nutritional medicine led to training in environmental medicine and then ayurveda, an Indian system of natural, holistic medicine. I integrated the best of this new knowledge into what I had already learned from thirty years of medical practice, nineteen of it holistic.

When Ken consulted me about his cancer-burdened body-mind, he had access to all of this integrated knowledge and experience. He made superb use of it.

Ken's healing affirmed the value of the path I had followed for the past eleven years and the good that had been redeemed from suffering and death. It became a part of my own healing and reinforced my determination to continue my quest.

Discovery

I cannot remember at what point during the 11 years between Andy's death and Ken's deliverance I first realized that the 100-year healthspan is our birthright from Nature. The awareness grew gradually from the periphery of my consciousness. By the autumn of 1995, the realization was clear. I sat down beside a brook that runs through our property and began to dictate this book.

I use Dr. Deepak Chopra's definition of health. Dr. Chopra said that so long as we have human bodies, we will experience both comfort and discomfort. In sickness, discomfort predominates. In health, comfort predominates. In perfect health, bliss predominates. In other words, what I had learned was that Nature intends for us to enjoy a state of being in which our comfort predominates over our discomfort until we are at least 100 years old.

With the realization that nature intends us to enjoy the 100-year healthspan came a state of cognitive dissonance: what I knew did not match what I saw. I had never seen or heard of anybody, in my lifetime, who had enjoyed a preponderance of comfort over discomfort until the age of 100. It was not until 1998 that I heard of Leila Denmark, M.D., a pediatrician, who celebrated her 100th birthday in February of that year. According to *the Atlanta Constitution* and the *Medical College of Georgia Magazine,* Dr. Denmark sees patients every day and still finds time to play golf. She said, "My health is perfect. I work every day. You have to eat right and love what you are doing. When people ask me when I am going to retire, I say, 'Check the obituaries.' ... The happiest time of my life was from the time I was born until now."

Those who have been checking the obituaries for news of Dr. Denmark's retirement must be getting rather bored. The same newspaper recently noted her 101st birthday—and that she is still going strong and caring for her patients.

It is important to understand that when I use Dr. Chopra's definition of health, I am not referring to physical comfort and discomfort alone. I practice holistic medicine, so I consider not only the physical level of life, but also the mental and spiritual levels. The Whole Self Diagram, in the Appendix, indicates how I see those three levels and their subdivisions. It is important to understand that comfort refers to more than the physical level because *physical* discomfort may sometimes predominate over physical comfort; yet the total comfort of the Whole Self may predominate over the physical discomfort due to the predominance of comfort on the mental and spiritual levels.

For example, a woman running a marathon may have a great preponderance of physical discomfort over comfort, but she might be experiencing so much emotional and spiritual fulfillment from the experience that her comfort on those higher levels overrode the physical discomfort. Her total comfort level would then predominate over her discomfort. On the other hand, had she chosen to stay home and lounge in the hammock that day, she would probably be comfortable physically. However, she might be so ashamed and disappointed in herself for failing to keep a commitment to herself that her mental discomfort overwhelmed her physical comfort, so that discomfort was predominant in her Whole Self. Please remember that when I refer to comfort and discomfort in the definition of health, it always refers to the Whole Self and not to only one level, such as the physical.

Evidence for the 100-year healthspan

One of the important functions of this book is to advance some evidence in support of the 100-year healthspan. As noted earlier, if you do not believe it is possible, you are unlikely to do the things that empower you to experience it. We present the following six lines of evidence for your consideration.

Growing younger

The workshop on crisis mastery had been intense. Most participants looked tired as they gathered their belongings and began to leave. Rosie, on the other hand, was animated and energetic as she chatted about her plans for continuing to assemble a print and tape library of works on natural healing. She intends it to be a resource for her section of the state. The strength of her voice, the sparkle in her eye, the spring in her step, and the healthy glow of her complexion surpassed that of other workshop participants half her age. Rosie is 75.

It was not always this way with Rosie. When she consulted me several years ago because of chronic, severe sinus infections and sore throat, she was so fatigued that she could hardly drag herself out of bed each morning. As I took her history, I learned that she had been depressed for as long as she could remember. She had anxiety, daytime drowsiness, and felt "stressed out." A holistic evaluation revealed that she had decreased thyroid system function of a type that is undetectable by blood tests but characterized by a low body temperature. Adrenal testing revealed a deficiency of two crucially important adrenal hormones, cortisol and DHEA. Digestive analysis showed hypochlorhydria (insufficient hydrochloric acid in the stomach). Her symptoms also suggested an imbalance of the subtle energy that the Chinese call *chi*. Her lifestyle was excessively stressful and out of balance. She wasn't experiencing enough mental quietness and peace to balance her intense activity as community activist and apartment complex manager.

Her holistic treatment program included interventions on biochemical, energy, and consciousness levels. The biochemical prescriptions included a multiple vitamin and mineral supplement, flax oil, vitamin C in the largest doses she could take without getting diarrhea, and tyrosine for depression. For the sinus infection and severe sore throat, I gave her infusions of vitamin C, magnesium, B complex, and B-12. For the energy imbalance, I referred her for craniosacral therapy with an osteopath who I knew was highly skilled and effective. Consciousness interventions included meditation and gaining knowledge about mind-body and energy medicine. Much of this she learned from the works of Deepak Chopra, M.D. and Caroline Myss, Ph.D. She modified her life style to reduce some of the occupational and political stress.

She responded to treatment with a complete recovery from chronic sinusitis and sore throats. Her lifelong depression improved and her anxiety, fatigue, drowsiness, and stressed out feeling almost disappeared. She told me that the things that helped her most were meditation, which gave her a much-needed experience of quiet alertness, thyroid supplementation with a thyroid hormone called T3, and adrenal support with cortisol.

In a recent follow up consultation she said, "I feel hopeful of living life free of pain and suffering in my old age. I'm looking forward to being able to leave off some of the pills I'm now taking. I now feel like I did when I was in my sixties. I feel much more secure knowing that if I do get an infection, there are natural remedies such as the vitamin C and the IV's, and I won't have to take drugs." I told Rosie that, as she continues to use her holistic program, I expected within another year or two she will be feeling like she did when she was in her fifties. As I watched her at the conclusion of the workshop, it appeared that the prediction had been fulfilled sooner than I had expected.

Rosie is one of many patients who has shown me that it is possible to reduce one's biological age while chronological age advances. This is one of the capabilities that makes the 100-year healthspan feasible.

Six converging lines

I gained the knowledge that nature's birthright to us human beings is the 100-year healthspan from the convergence of six different lines of evidence:

1. Experiences gained from more than 40 years of medical practice

2. The conclusions of gerontologists about the potential length of the human life span

3. Observations from Abkhasia and other long-lived cultures

4. A rapidly growing body of scientific evidence that behavioral and other natural interventions can retard or reverse biological aging.

5. Expansion of knowledge and use of new and old healing technologies at a rate unprecedented in history. Large numbers and widespread availability of talented practitioners and teachers synergize this expansion.

6. Rapid and extensive dissemination of this knowledge by the new technologies of mass communication systems such as the Internet. This fortunate synergism of circumstances creates the potential for higher levels and longer duration of health than humankind has ever known before.

Clinical experience

In my practice of holistic medicine, I encourage my patients to act on three important levels of life, mental, physical, and spiritual, in order to achieve their 100-year healthspan. Not every patient chooses to do this. Many patients believe the cultural prescription, "Feeling ill? Pop a pill!" Others, and their numbers are growing each year, know that the culture is not prescribing the best course for fulfillment of health potential. This growing group of patients wants the information, inspiration, and guidance to take control of their own lives and particularly their own health. They are not only willing, but also hungry, to know how to create balance and harmony within their body-minds. These patients have taught me much. As the years have come and gone and my repertoire of natural interventions has steadily expanded, I am able to teach my patients increasingly effective interventions. They are responding by achieving improvements in health and performance that were inconceivable a decade ago.

Louis, 76 and retired, consulted me because he wished to be free of the necessity of taking heart medicine. He had consulted his physician when he began to have shortness of breath while climbing the hill from his mailbox to his house. He learned that he had congestive heart failure for which he should take some medicine. Shortness of breath stopped, but he wished to improve his heart function by natural means. After hearing that I practice holistic medicine, he consulted me.

From Louis's history, I learned that he drank too much coffee and not enough water, ate too many carbohydrates and not enough protein, and did not know how to experience the mind-state of quiet alertness. We worked out a holistic recovery program that addressed each of these imbalances and included Coenzyme Q-10 100 mg twice daily, together with other supplements to strengthen heart function.

Louis returned two months later looking 15 years younger and glowing with health. When I asked about shortness of breath, he looked surprised. He had forgotten about it. That is always a good sign. He said he had experienced none since his first consultation.

We agreed that after another two months on his holistic program, he would ask his heart doctor about reducing the medicine. I asked Louis, "When you first consulted me how old did you feel?"

Louis looked thoughtful, then smiled, and said, "Late middle age."

"Now how old do you feel?" I asked.

Louis' smile widened. "Younger than that—middle age," he replied.

He was able to stop taking the heart medicine without further trouble with shortness of breath.

Seeing Louis, Rosie, and many other people who have already attained advanced age and made dramatic improvements in the way they feel and function, has expanded my horizon to the point that I now know the 100-year healthspan is feasible for many people in modern western culture. In fact, for the first time in history, I believe it is feasible for the majority of people in the western world.

The conclusion of gerontologists

Gerontologists are scientists who study the aging process. There is now a consensus among them that human beings are genetically endowed to live 115 to 150 years. I just do not hear any further debate about this. It seems reasonable that, if it is encoded in our DNA for us to live at least 115 years, we should be able to stay healthy at least one hundred of those. Actually, knowing what I now know, seeing what I have seen, and hearing what I have heard from my patients and friends, it does not seem unreasonable that a person could enjoy complete mental, physical and spiritual well being until the day she dies. We write about several examples in the *Epilogue*. In addition to those, I have heard of other contemporaries who died, "dropped their bodies" as the Indians say, without illness or trauma. A friend told me that Buckminster Fuller, the architect and philosopher, sat beside his wife's bed until she died, then rested his head on the bed, and died.

I have heard enough of these stories to believe that human beings can cultivate the ability to die, to drop the body, without illness or trauma, in the time, place and manner of their own choosing, because they have completed the purpose for which they came into this life. This is a graceful and fitting conclusion to a 100-year healthspan. It is also part of our birthright from nature. Not everyone will choose to drop his body on the day after his 100th birthday. Some people will need longer for mission fulfillment—110, 120, maybe 150 years. Some will not need that long. The important things are the freedom to choose and the power to execute the choice.

It has been said that everybody has to die of something. While that is probably true, what one dies of obviously does not have to be sickness or violence. As these accounts make clear, one may choose to die of the fulfillment of one's life purpose and the desire to see what comes next. When Justice Oliver William Holmes was dying, his last words were, "And now, the great adventure!"

Abkhasia

The next line of evidence is that there are already cultures in the world where many people achieve the 100-year healthspan. The most notable of these is a province in central Russia called Abkhasia. Abkhasia has been called the longevity belt. It has attracted researchers from all over the world because of the remarkable healthspan of its people.

Abkhasia lies between the Caspian and the Black seas and includes the highest mountain range in Russia. Abkhasians frequently live past 100 years. On their 100th birthdays, many are vigorous, active, productive, and zestful. Research has shown that their remarkable health spans are not due to genetics, because they are a genetically diverse people, or due to climate which varies from subtropical to high alpine. Dr. Deepak Chopra, in *Ageless Body, Timeless Mind*, has written a detailed

discussion of this region and its people. I encourage you to read
that book.

Chopra's conclusion is that the long healthspan of the
Abkhasians is multifactorial. He believes that one of the most
important factors is the national attitude toward the long living.
There are no old people in Abkhasia, but there are plenty of the
long living. Achieving longevity has the same status in Abkhasia
that achieving financial wealth has in this country. The long living, particularly those who are physically active, are considered
glamorous. They are envied and given places of honor in social
events such as parades, where they ride horseback. Horseback
riding and horse racing are the national pastimes of Abkhasia.
Those who perform acrobatics on horseback are the superstars
of the Abkhasian sporting world.

Another national pastime is duping foreigners with tall tales
about Abkhasian longevity. Researchers have learned that they
need to carefully document the claims of the Abkhasians lest
they fall victim to the Abkhasian delight in fooling foreigners.
Even after deflation of exaggerated claims about longevity, the
Abkhasians still demonstrate the feasibility of the 100-year
healthspan.

The Abkhasian diet is no doubt a factor in their longevity.
They eat unprocessed, locally grown food and they eat it fresh.
When meat is to be served to guests, the guests are shown the
animal before it is slaughtered. There are no leftovers in
Abkhasia. Food is discarded if it is not eaten at the meal in which
it was cooked. Ayurveda and advanced American nutrition also
highly esteem fresh food and advise against using leftovers.

I can speak from experience about fresh food. I remember
visiting a friend on a farm. I happened to be there at dinnertime
(midday, of course). My friend's mother scooped up a chicken,
which happened to be walking across the back porch, wrung its
neck over the porch rail, and plucked it. Once the chicken was in
the skillet, she made biscuits and gravy. Within an hour of the
time the chicken made its transition into its next existence, not

without trauma and violence unfortunately, we were eating its remains. Thus, we fulfilled Dr. Abram Hoffer's admonition that food should be eaten alive or recently alive. The Abkhasians enjoy these benefits and pleasures every day. In addition to subsisting mainly on fresh vegetables and dairy products, they also eat a small amount of meat and some grain.

Their quantity of food consumption is low by western standards. They probably consume 1500 to 2000 calories a day while engaging in an active lifestyle. Most of their work is outdoors in the fields, and it is not unusual for them to walk twenty miles a day. Not surprisingly, most of them have a lean physique.

The outdoor environment in which they spend most of their time is relatively pure, since the region is agricultural and not industrialized.

Those who have studied the Abkhasians have been impressed with how much they appear to be in harmony with nature. The rhythms and cycles of their lives are essentially the rhythms and cycle of nature. In his commentary on the Abkhasians, Dr. Chopra observes that their culture has programmed them to live in the healthy manner that we in the western world are struggling to attain. They do not have to overcome the cultural pressure toward abusive lifestyles.

There are a few other cultures, most notably the tribes in the high Andes, that have achieved extraordinary longevity and healthspan. The long living in the high Andes are esteemed for their ability to run long distances. Soaring Eagle, a Native American personal trainer who has developed a holistic healthspan program, told me that their idea for a marathon is to run non-stop for three days and two nights. When some of them accepted an invitation to run a marathon in the US, they were astonished and confused when the race was over after only 26 miles. AT&T has not penetrated that area and the news travels at the speed of feet. It is generally acknowledged that the long living are the best at long running.

Knowledge of these cultures in which the 100-year healthspan is the norm is reassuring to us that the 100-year healthspan is indeed a feasible human experience.

USA demographics

From 1980 to 1990 the ninety-five to ninety-nine year age group had the highest percentage increase in the population: ninety-six percent. Statistics from the Census Bureau and the Social Security Administration, quoted in *Ageless Body, Timeless Mind,* tell us that we are winning the battle for longevity in this country. The number of centenarians in 1993 was estimated by the Census Bureau to be around 36,000. That number is expected to double before the year 2000. Social Security Administration figures, probably more reliable than the Census Bureau's, indicate that one person in ten thousand is 100 years old or more. In Iowa, it is even better: one in approximately four thousand. Utah has only one in approximately twenty thousand.

While we are obviously winning the battle for longevity, we are not winning it for the 100-year healthspan. Anthony Smith wrote in *The Body,* "Put at its crudest, the advances of medicine are enabling more and more of us to achieve senility". According to a Center for Disease Control study of several thousand people who died in 1983 between the ages of sixty-five and seventy-four, only twenty percent were "fully functional." That meant they could dress themselves, walk, eat, go to the toilet and bathe without assistance. Ten percent were "severely restricted", meaning that they required assistance with three or more of these functions.

I would like to propose a more generous description of "fully functional." Carl's granddaddy, whose last day on earth I will describe in the Epilogue, was fully functional. So is an Air Force general who runs up three flights of steps to his office every day, teaches five classes and celebrates each birthday by going to the infirmary for a flight physical. After passing the physical he goes out on the flight line, climbs in an F-15 and takes off.

If this does not sound very surprising for an Air Force general, it is because I did not tell you that he is retired and is eighty-six years old. His name is Robert L. Scott. He was an ace in the American Volunteer Group, the "Flying Tigers", fighting the Japanese in China, just before the outbreak of World War II. He is the author of two books, *God Is My Co-Pilot,* and *The Day I Owned the Sky.* General Scott's activities, recorded in *The Albany Herald,* qualify him for my definition of "fully functional". He is well on his way to enjoying the 100 year healthspan. A patient of mine, who enjoyed talking with General Scott at a reception, said that he told her that fulfilling his purpose in life (teaching the importance of air power in maintaining world peace) is fundamentally important to him. "When a person stops being useful, it is time to die." Perhaps another way of saying that would be "When one has fulfilled one's purpose in life it is time to own the sky."

Scientific research

Substantial scientific research supports the concept of the 100-year healthspan. Much of it has been conducted on people who are doing Transcendental Meditation (TM). One of the first papers to be published reported what happens to the metabolic rate when one is practicing TM. The metabolic rate measures how fast the body burns oxygen to produce energy. Metabolic rates are always compared to the basal metabolic rate (B.M.R.), which is the rate at which the body burns oxygen when lying quietly in bed after first awakening in the morning. When you are active, your metabolic rate is higher than your B.M.R. When you have been sleeping for several hours it is lower—about eighteen percent lower. The researcher who did this study found that after a few minutes of practicing TM, the metabolic rate was thirty percent below basal.

This discovery led to the question, "If one substantially lowers her metabolic rate regularly, twice a day, might this retard the aging process?" A study was done to determine the biological age of meditators. To understand this research you need to know that you have two ages: your chronological age and your biological age. Some people have three ages: chronological, biological, and the one they tell when asked in social situations. You already know about your chronological age; the calendar tells you that. Your biological age is your functional age. It is how much you can do physically and how efficiently your physiology works compared to that of the average person in our culture. There can be a great difference between chronological age and biological age. A person with a chronological age of twenty may be biologically forty—and vice versa. The research on the biological age of meditators showed that those who had been meditating less than five years were, on the average, six years younger biologically than their chronological age. Meditators of more than five years practice averaged twelve years younger than their chronological age. One woman was a full twenty years younger biologically than she was chronologically. Do you like the idea of being biologically forty years old when the calendar says you are sixty?

We are not intending to imply here that TM is the best way to meditate to assist one in living the 100-year healthspan. More studies have been done on TM than the other meditative techniques, partly because one pays a substantial amount of money to learn TM. The TM movement, therefore, has more resources to fund studies. There are not yet enough studies to compare TM with other forms of meditation, such as Zen.

The next question was, "Do people who are biologically younger than their chronological age get sick less frequently than those who are biologically and chronologically the same age, or biologically older than their chronological age?" Research has been done on that, too. It found that meditators, on the average, had about half the health care utilization of matched-control non-meditators. This effect was smallest in the under-twenty age group and largest in the over-forty.

Meditators over forty had about sixty-five percent less health care usage than those who didn't meditate. When you consider that it is the over-forty age group that is bankrupting the American health care system, this becomes an interesting observation. Even more interesting was the breakout of the incidence of cancer and heart disease among meditators. These two diseases are the leading causes of death in the US. Meditators had eighty percent less hospitalization for heart disease than non-meditators and about fifty percent less hospitalization for tumors including cancer. Clearly, there is evidence that what you do can have a major favorable impact on the quality of your health and the duration of your healthspan.

Robert Herron did the following research for his Ph.D. dissertation. Dr. Harri Sharma reported it in his book, *Freedom from Disease*. This study examined health care expenditures for Canadians for three years before and three years after they began to do Transcendental Meditation. After they began to meditate, their health care costs decreased ten percent a year for a total of 30 percent over three years. The third of the population that were the heaviest users of health care had an 18 percent per year decrease with a total decrease of 54 percent in three years. The elderly had a 19 percent per year decrease with a total decrease of 57 percent. Clearly, just one intervention can have a powerful, highly significant effect on the need for medical treatment.

What about combining two or more interventions? Would there be a synergistic effect? There has not been much research on this yet, but there is one interesting study on what happens to health care utilization when an ayurvedic rejuvenation and detoxification procedure called panchakarma is added to meditation. It was found that people doing both things had 84 percent less hospitalization than matched controls.

Rapid expansion of knowledge and availability of healing technologies

The last decade has brought the most rapid expansion of useful and available knowledge and technologies for improving health that humankind has experienced within recorded history. Some of these interventions have been known for a long time but have only recently become generally available. Some examples are acupuncture, acupressure, tai chi, chi gong, therapeutic touch, ayurveda, cognitive behavioral therapy, naturopathy, and homeopathy. Some technologies are only now emerging: psychoneuroimmunology, the human genome project, energy anatomy techniques of Dr. Caroline Myss, wound healing and tissue regeneration technologies of Dr. Bart Flick and others, Whole Self Balancing as presented in this book and in *The Life We Are Given*, by Leonard and Murphy.

Whole Self Balancing is a systematic and harmonious integration of several natural ways of enhancing health. It creates a synergy among its components that is more powerful than the sum of the parts. We believe that it offers a substantial enhancement of the probability of attaining the 100-year healthspan. It is part of the reason that this attainment is feasible for many for the first time in history. Together, this broad array of interventions offers something for everyone who seeks safe, natural, effective ways of enhancing health. The number of such persons is legion.

One of the demographic hallmarks of the baby boomer generation is a strong desire and determination to take charge of and responsibility for their own health. There is the understanding that this is possible only through natural means, including healthy lifestyle, not through drugs and surgery. To serve this huge market there is a multitude of practitioners and teachers, many of whom are talented and effective. Some outstanding examples include Deepak Chopra, MD, Andrew Weil, MD, Julian Whitaker, MD, Caroline Myss, Ph.D. and Wayne Dyer, Ph.D.

A Criticism of the Concept

When we presented the concept of the 100-year healthspan in an Elderhostel program, a participant who was a neurologist immediately denounced it as absurd, irresponsible and harmful.

She said that attaining the 100-year healthspan is obviously impossible, so to create that expectation is to set people up for failure, disappointment and harm: "Send them down the tubes," as she put it. My response was that for the first time in history the 100-year healthspan *is* possible for large numbers of people because of two factors.

The first we have already mentioned: knowledge of healing modalities has increased to a critical mass, as new technologies are developed and old ones rediscovered. This makes possible the attainment of levels of health unprecedented in history. This knowledge is available to masses of people worldwide through the Internet and other modern communication technologies. The information superhighway has revolutionized the speed and density of information exchange, creating possibilities that are unique in human history. The combination of these two factors has created a new group consciousness in a significantly large subset of the population that supports the achievement of levels of health and well-being never before reached.

The second factor is that I agree with Wayne Dyer's advice to accept no limitations, because no one knows what he can actually accomplish until he makes his best effort. To accept a limitation is to be bound by it. "Argue for your limitations and they are yours," says Dr. Stephen Covey. To assume that the 100-year healthspan, or anything else, is impossible makes its attainment virtually impossible. Thoreau wrote, "Men eventually hit only what they aim at. Therefore they had better aim high though they fail immediately." In the years I was doing target practice, I knew that I would not always hit the bulls eye; but I always aimed for it anyway. I knew that I would hit it more often and always come closer to it than if I aimed below the target. Aiming for the bulls eye carried a higher risk of disappointment, but it also produced higher performance.

In the ensuing discussion, I recalled Chopra's comments about health, comfort, and discomfort. As you may recall, he wrote that as long as we have human bodies we will experience both comfort and discomfort. In sickness, discomfort predominates. In health, comfort predominates. In perfect health, bliss predominates. Since some discomfort is a given regardless of one's state of health, it seems desirable to arrange to have a predominance of comfort. The interventions presented in this book are designed to accomplish that as they support the attainment of the 100-year healthspan.

For these reasons, I know that advocating for attainment of the 100-year healthspan is neither absurd, irresponsible, nor harmful. The other physician maintained her position. I thanked her for challenging me to consider more carefully what I am doing. Because of considering and responding to her criticism, I now proceed with more confidence, conviction, and power to fulfill my mission.

If It Is Possible, Why Isn't Everyone Doing It?

Very few people are claiming their birthright of the 100 year healthspan because of several formidable challenges: we live in a degraded environment, eat a degraded food supply and live abusive lifestyles in a culture dominated by superstition and ignorance.

In the next chapter, we will consider these hazards in some detail.

Chapter 2

DREAM DESTROYERS and BIRTHRIGHT BURGLARS

"If you are sitting on three tacks, you have an environmental problem —you may be living in a tacky environment"

—The Third Tacks Law of Sidney M. Baker, M.D.

If the 100-year healthspan is nature's birthright to human beings, why are so few people claiming it? There are plenty of reasons. Modern life is full of hazards. Fortunately, for every hazard there is at least one countermeasure. We will consider the latter in detail in the second section of this book, Knowledge for Claiming Your Birthright. First, we will briefly describe the hazards. They include a perilously polluted environment, degraded food supply, disease-inducing diets, abusive lifestyles, immune suppression, dangerous mutations of viruses and bacteria, superstition, and ignorance. Since most people are somewhat aware of most of these hazards, I will try to be brief in this chapter, the sooner to move on to the helpful, powerful knowledge in Section Two.

A PERILOUSLY POLLUTED ENVIRONMENT

We have all participated in the poisoning of our planet, our Mother Earth. We have dumped so many tons of poisonous chemicals on her that she is sick and can no longer nurture her offspring as she intended and wishes. Because of this irresponsible behavior by most of us, we are all sitting on at least three tacks. The reason that not all of us are sick yet is that some people have tougher butts than others. Every butt has its unique tack tolerance, but either we clean up the environmental mess or we will *all* be sick eventually. Many people already are.

Ever hear of sick building syndrome? It is real—and it is not the building that is sick. The National Cancer Institute estimates that toxic chemicals cause ninety percent of cancers. Thousands of people with respiratory disease die every year of air pollution in our cities. Even the once-pristine forests of the Great Smokies National Park, the Skyline Drive, and the Blue Ridge Parkway are dying of air pollution. More and more people are becoming chemically sensitive, reacting to even minute amounts of chemicals in air, food and water because their detoxification abilities have been overwhelmed by the flood of toxic chemicals that come with eating, drinking and breathing in the late 20th century.

Electromagnetic radiation is undetectable by the senses but can be deadly. A colleague and friend asked me to see his teenage son, who was complaining of fatigue, weakness, and muscle pain. It sounded like chronic fatigue syndrome that I expected would respond to some intravenous infusions of magnesium and vitamins. When I saw the boy, I was alarmed to see that he looked very sick. He was so weak he could hardly stand, his muscles were so tender he could barely tolerate my touching them, and he was pale. He said that not only his muscles, but also his joints, hurt. His throat was severely inflamed. I asked his mother to take him immediately to an emergency room. Later that night she phoned to say that a blood count had revealed an extremely high white count of a type that was consistent with acute leukemia. The boy's parents were horrified and terrified.

After securing the best medical treatment they could find, the father set out to discover what might have caused the leukemia. As part of the investigation, he retained an environmental engineer to survey the house for toxic environmental influences.

The engineer discovered that the electromagnetic field in the boy's room was 5,000 times the safe level. This toxic electrical field was created by a television, a powerful sound system and infrared and ultraviolet lighting crowded into a small space. The association between strong electrical fields and leukemia in children is well documented, but furiously denied by electrical companies. During the cold war, the Soviets microwaved the U.S. Embassy, producing an electromagnetic field that caused fatigue and headache in the people working there.

Noise pollution also takes its toll. Human beings need intervals of silence and certainly not the constant high-decibel background noise of city life. Noise pollution is a significant stress that adds to the total stress load of most people in this country. The total load of overstress is a major factor in shortening the healthspan.

UNSAFE WATER

USA Today published an article on the decline in safety of the water supply, quoting from a report published by the American Academy of Microbiology, "A Global Decline In Microbiological Safety Of Water. A Call for Action." The report cited data from the US and international health agencies. According to this report, pollution of the water by chemicals and metals causes disease, but eighty percent of disease caused by drinking water is due to microbes, such as bacteria, viruses, and parasites. Many outbreaks of disease result from water that comes out of faucets at home. These outbreaks often go unrecognized. The report recommends drinking bottled water or using home water treatment programs as a short-term solution. However, is bottled water safe? Studies have shown that, because it is not regulated, bottled water—including Perrier and Evian, can and often does contain more pollutants than tap water. For that reason, I recommend filtering water at home.

In 1991, the Centers for Disease Control identified 554 disease outbreaks affecting 136,000 people caused by contaminated drinking water. Between 1986 and 1992, one third of public water systems violated US standards for water purity. In 1993 an outbreak of Cryptosporidium disease, water borne, made 400,000 sick and killed 110 in Milwaukee. In ten years, the incidence of disease due to contaminated water is up 250 percent.

Can we look to the federal government for help? We wonder. Legislation to address the problem has been introduced in the US Congress. It is supposed to raise standards for water purity. We have seen a press release by a private environmental organization saying that the legislation actually lowers standards for water purity. I hope this is not true, but it is consistent with governmental response dealing with social problems. For example, when the decline in the quality of education was reflected in declining SAT scores, the response was to make the test easier. When surveys revealed that the majority of the US population received less than the recommended daily allowance of vitamin B6, the recommendation by a committee of the National Academy of Science was to lower the recommended daily allowance. After all, we wouldn't want to alarm people or make them think there is anything wrong with the Standard American Diet. Never mind the fact that B6 is essential for healthy immune and nervous system function and detoxification processes in the body.

I think the bottom line is that people who are interested in experiencing the 100 year healthspan should assume that tap water is pure enough for washing the car and flushing the toilet, but no longer fit for human consumption. In Part 2 we will address the vital issue of what to do about it.

DEGRADED FOOD SUPPLY

Something funny happened to your food on the way to the dinner table. In fact, several funny things happened to it. Better have a box of tissues handy before you read this. If you do not laugh, you may cry. These are some things that I learned from one of my mentors, Jonathan V. Wright, M.D. Jonathan is an incredibly bright, hardworking nutritional physician who does his homework. He is also a gifted writer and a valiant, effective warrior (ask the FDA) for the cause of freedom, particularly freedom of choice in healthcare. His personal research library, now computerized, includes over 35,000 medical journal articles dating from 1920 to the present. He has published several books on nutritional medicine and one on natural hormone replacement. His most recent title is *Maximize Your Vitality and Potency for Men Over 40*. He also edits a monthly newsletter. All are written for the consumer and packed with useful information about nutrition and natural healing. See *Resources* in the Appendix for details and his web page address.

Jonathan reads a lot. He has read USDA reports on mineral analysis done on food grown by US agribusiness. Every few years the FDA tested samples of a variety of produce for mineral content. With every test, the mineral content decreased. This was happening probably because the food was grown on land that was treated like a strip mine. There were heavy applications of chemical fertilizers, with little or no attention to replacing humus and the trace minerals that are necessary for human health but not for plant growth. The declining levels of trace minerals in the American food supply are not good news for health, since these minerals are necessary for health and good immune function.

The problem is made worse by the hybridization of food-producing plants. Plant geneticists working for agribusiness have been breeding plants to produce fruit and vegetables that have attractive appearance and long shelf life. I have heard that the dream of these geneticists is to breed a tomato plant that will produce tomatoes that can be dropped seventeen feet onto concrete without bruising. My recent experience with commercially produced tomatoes is that they are close to fulfillment of this dream. Maybe, once they have accomplished this goal, they will go on to hybridize plants that will produce tomatoes that can be used in National League batting practice during the season and then, after the World Series, crated and taken off to the supermarkets to go on the produce counters.

Unfortunately, when plants are bred to produce fruits and vegetables for great appearance and long shelf life, the flavor and nutritional value usually decrease. If you want to see what we mean, for flavor try an organically grown vine-ripened tomato and then one bought off the produce counter. Be fair: Do it blindfolded. There will be as much difference in the nutritional value, which you cannot taste, as there will in the flavor. How do I know? Bob Smith was once the director of Doctors' Data, a reference laboratory that did a lot of work for nutritional and environmental physicians in the US. As a professional hobby, for ten years he compared the mineral content of agribusiness produce with organically grown food. His conclusion at the end of this study was that the organically grown food had ten times the mineral value of the agribusiness product.

What does this mean for the 100-year healthspan? It means that if you eat commercially produced food and you do not supplement with vitamins and minerals, you are not playing with a full deck. Your biochemistry will not be functioning well enough to give you the best chance to claim nature's birthright.

Unfortunately, the sad story does not end here. After being hybridized for great looks and low nutrient content and grown on land that has been abused and depleted of nutrients, the food is liberally poisoned. I also learned from Jonathan that the EPA did market basket surveys for herbicide and pesticide contamination of food. In the next to the last study, eighty percent of the food in the market basket was contaminated. In the last one, it was 100 percent. We have not heard of any tests since then. Maybe the EPA decided there was no point in testing anymore because things had gotten as bad as they could get. Unfortunately, they had not. As insects mutate to become resistant to pesticides and plant resistance to disease and insects decline because of hybridization, more and stronger pesticides have to be used. I think we have to assume that the intensity of contamination of food is steadily increasing. Want to know why pesticides kill bugs quicker than they kill people? It's because people are bigger. Because the poisons on and in your food do not kill you as quickly as they did some of the bugs does not mean that they are not harming your health.

However, even that is not the end of the story. After the food is grown on mineral-depleted land by plants that have been bred for appearance rather than nutritional value and then poisoned, it is "partitioned". That is the food processing industry's term for taking out the parts of the food that are most life supporting. Why would anyone want to do that? Because the most nutritious part of the food nourishes not only people, but also bacteria and fungi. These make the food spoil sooner. This means short shelf life.

If you want to make the most profit on food, you can not have short shelf life. Therefore, you take out the most nutritious part, like taking wheat germ out of wheat flour. With the wheat germ gone, flour will keep practically forever. Since it has lost most of its vitamin and mineral value, it is "enriched". This means that eight vitamins and minerals are put back into the flour after eighteen have been taken out. This is like someone robbing you at gunpoint on a dark street on a winter night, taking your money and clothes and then, at the last minute, taking pity on your shivering embarrassment, giving back your underwear and bus fare home and telling you that he has enriched you.

Alas, there is more to this sad saga. Most of the food in the supermarket, on the shelves along the aisles, has been dead for a long time. Abram Hoffer, MD, one of the pioneers in modern nutritional medicine, advises us to eat food that is alive or recently alive. He's not recommending gulping down live goldfish. When Genevieve goes to the garden, picks lettuce, and uses it to make our dinner salad, we are eating food that is alive. When I pick lima beans during the morning, Genevieve cooks them for dinner, and we eat them less than three hours after they came off the plants, that is recently alive. Alive and recently alive food is a good idea because it has enzymes that don't last long after the food dies. Enzymes were necessary for the plant's life and they enhance yours, if you get them. Foods in those pretty boxes that have a shelf life measured in months and years do not have many enzymes left. Even rats will not eat some of it. A wise nutritional physician has said that if rats and bacteria will not eat the food, you should not either.

There is one more thing to know about this nutrient-depleted, poisoned, partitioned, long-dead food. It is super-abundant. There is an abundance of it and most people eat too much of it. The situation is similar to the story about people in the old west who depended on buffalo meat to get them through the winter. There was a community meeting, and the announcement, "There's good news and bad news. The bad news is that the buffalo hunt was a failure, and we don't have any buffalo meat to get us through the winter. All we have is buffalo chips. The good news is, there's plenty of them."

If you are going to be eating food of the quality described above, you are better off eating a little of it than a lot of it. Even if you are eating nutritious food, you are better off eating a little than a lot. How you eat and how much you eat are as important as what you eat. The way most of us do it in the western world is not supportive of the 100-year healthspan.

TOO MUCH OF THE WRONG FOOD, IN THE WRONG BALANCE, EATEN AT THE WRONG TIME, IN THE WRONG WAY

It is a basic principle of nutritional medicine that one will be healthier eating a small amount of a poor diet than overeating a good diet. This is a paradox. The difference between a paradox and a contradiction is that there is a key that explains the paradox and reconciles it. There is no reconciliation of a contradiction. The key to reconciling the nutritional paradox is actually three keys. The first key is that if you eat too much you get fat. Being fat is one of the two risk factors for every known degenerative disease. Three hundred thousand people in the US die every year because of obesity. The other universal risk factor, in case you are wondering, is smoking. Fat smokers generally don't have to wait long for one or more degenerative diseases to appear.

The second key is free radicals, oxygen molecules that have lost an electron. Eating stimulates the production of free radicals. You have to have free radicals to digest and assimilate your food, produce energy, and protect against disease. You have to have enough, but there is such a thing as too many free radicals. When you have too many, when they get through doing the necessary things for your health, they start ripping and tearing your cell membranes, damaging your tissues and preparing the way for disease. Overeating causes the overproduction of free radicals.

The third key is excessively high blood sugar and insulin. When your blood sugar goes too high and stays high for long periods, you start making AGES (advanced glycosylation end products). AGES are one of the two basic factors in rapid aging. The other is excessive free radical production. You see, it is very efficient: all you have to do to get too much of both is overeat. AGES age you by cross-linking the protein in your tissues with glucose molecules. This makes your tissues leathery and increasingly rigid—not the way you want them to be for complete mental and physical well being when you are 100 years old. Therefore, while a poor diet is not a desirable thing, it is generally less of a birthright burglar than excessive amounts of a good diet. If you overeat a poor diet, you are entertaining a big birthright burglar.

How much food is enough? Enough is the amount that maintains your lean body mass at about seventy-five percent and your body fat at about twenty-five percent if you are female and about eighty-five percent and fifteen percent if you are male. Enough also gives you abundant energy and, if you balance protein, carbohydrate and fat appropriately, keeps you from being hungry, and from craving carbohydrates. How many calories that amounts to depends on your lean body mass and your activity level. Two people with the same lean body mass will vary widely in their calorie requirements, depending on whether or not they are engaged in strenuous physical activity several hours a day or pursuing the couch potato lifestyle. In Part II, we will consider how to calculate your calorie requirements precisely in order to have a pleasing, healthy body composition, plenty of energy and freedom from food cravings. You probably will not be surprised to hear that most Americans eat too much. Americans are the fattest people on earth.

The current dietary wisdom is that the way to avoid overweight is to reduce fat and eat more carbohydrates. This has been the prevailing opinion for the past decade. During that time, the incidence of obesity has doubled in children and adolescents and has increased about thirty-five percent in adults. This should not be surprising. When agribusiness wants to fatten cattle, it feeds them lots of low-fat, high carbohydrate grain. The cattle obligingly fatten right up, particularly when their activities are limited. People are no different. One day, the nutritional establishment will catch on and the low fat, low protein, high carbohydrate prescription will change. You don't have to wait. If you are going for the 100-year healthspan, you can not afford to wait. We have already talked about how commercially produced food is the wrong thing. Now you know why eating it in the wrong amount is a health hazard. The story goes on.

In the Standard American Diet, appropriately abbreviated SAD, the ratio of protein, carbohydrate, and fat is out of balance. There is insufficient protein and too much carbohydrate and fat. For a fascinating and enlightening discussion of this, read *The Zone*, by Barry Sears, Ph.D. The most important result of the imbalance in favor of carbohydrates at the expense of protein is the overproduction of powerful tissue hormones called series two eicosanoids. These eicosanoids cause inflammation, excessive blood clotting, and free radical activity. The free radicals and accelerated clotting are bad enough, but these proinflammatory eicosanoids also cause disturbances of neurotransmitters that can cause depression, anxiety, agitation, brain fog, and excessive hunger. If you want to feel what we are talking about, eat a big pasta meal and notice how you feel two hours later. Particularly, notice how sharp your mind is two hours later. *The Zone* tells you how to get the correct balance of protein, carbohydrate, and fat. That gives you the correct balance of tissue hormones. Then you feel surprisingly well mentally and physically for hours after you eat.

So much for the wrong balance; what about eating it the wrong way? Ayurveda, the traditional Indian natural, holistic system of health care, long ago discovered that digestion is best when one eats in a relaxed, quiet, attractive environment and concentrates on enjoying every bite of food. Contrast this to the American way, in which food is generally eaten fast, at best in a noisy restaurant, at worst at one's desk, in one's car or during a business conference. This way of eating is a great blessing to gastroenterologists, because it guarantees them full employment. It is no blessing to you, because it reduces your chances of enjoying the 100-year healthspan.

Another devastator of good digestion is drinking ice cold beverages during a meal. Digestion depends on enzymes, and enzymes depend on a normal body temperature for optimum functioning. Ice water, iced tea, or cold beer definitely are not body temperature, or optimum enzyme temperature. Nevertheless, the American way is often to drink something ice cold with meals, even when the temperature outside is also ice cold.

The last wrong is the wrong time. Most people eat their biggest meal at night. Another discovery of ayurveda is that digestion is strongest when the sun is straight overhead. Does it make sense to give the digestive system its main work for the day when it is strongest? Eat a big meal late at night and we promise you maldigestion. The insidious thing is that if you have been maldigesting for years you may not even realize that it is happening.

Recently a patient told me that, until she started feeling so much better because of using the Healthspan Program, she had not realized how bad she had felt. It had been so many years since she had experienced abundant energy that she had forgotten it was possible. Nancy Sinatra sang, "I've been down so long it looks like up to me."

Well, thank goodness, that concludes the description of a birthright burglar named Malnutrition the American Way. You now have some valuable clues about using nutrition to maximize the probability of a long healthspan. You will get more detailed and interesting instructions in Section II. Now let us look at another dream destroyer called abusive lifestyles.

ABUSIVE LIFESTYLES

A man in his late forties was sitting in my consulting room to see what I could tell him about nutritional approaches to improving the quality of whatever life he had left. He had been told that he had liver cancer that had spread widely throughout his body. He was about to start chemotherapy, although that was unlikely to do more than buy him a few months of life. As I took his history, I learned that for years he had been feeling overburdened with teaching responsibilities at the college where he was on the faculty. Driven by fear of losing his job, he had agreed to teach several more classes each day than professors are supposed to teach. This had left him no time for research and writing, which he believes are important to fulfilling his purpose in life. He said, "It's really a relief to have this cancer. Now I finally have time for me."

Bernie Siegel, MD, in his wonderful book, *Love Medicine and Miracles*, talks about how often people who suddenly find they have a life threatening disease or who get into a severely disabling accident, then discover meaning and purpose in their lives. This leads many of them to say they are glad they have the disease or had the accident. Dr. Siegel comments on how sad and unnecessary it is that it takes such a catastrophe to enable a person to find meaning and purpose in life. That it does take such a crisis is a tribute to the power of what Chopra calls "the hypnosis of social conditioning."

Our culture is powerful in controlling what we think, say, and do. Educational psychologists estimate that by the time we reach adulthood, we have been subjected to 25,000 hours of social conditioning by our parents, teachers, acquaintances, and the media. We give society a pair of powerful conditioning tools with which to work on us: fear and greed. For most people, the two most powerful motivators are pain and fear. Actually, this comes down to pain because fear ultimately is the fear of experiencing pain of one kind or another. Society has convincing ways of saying, "If you don't fill these expectations, you are going to feel pain."

The other powerful motivator is greed: greed for power, approval, money, and security. Society is able to deliver all of the above except security, at least for limited intervals. It can never deliver security, but it can give the illusion of security, which is what most of us choose to settle for. There is a wonderful story in the New Testament about the farmer who had a fabulous bumper crop. His land produced so much that he had to tear down his barns and build bigger ones. At the end of the harvest, when his big barns were filled to capacity, he lay down to sleep saying to himself that at last he was secure. That night the Lord came to him and said, "You fool. Tonight your soul is required of you."

With its formidable tools of fear and greed, culture is likely to be able to drive most people most of the time into abusive lifestyles. An abusive lifestyle is one that creates imbalance within the individual's body-mind and between the individual and the rest of nature. Some frequent, culturally driven abusive lifestyles include

- too much work and not enough play
- too much of being a spectator and not enough of being a participant
- too much television and not enough creative mental activity
- too much eating and too little exercise
- too much competition and not enough cooperation

- too much loneliness and not enough companionship
- insufficient sleep

These imbalances are mortal enemies of the 100-year healthspan and represent an important part of the reason that the enjoyment of nature's birthright is pathetically rare. Suggestions for creating balance in each of these areas are included in the following chapters of this book.

The next hazard is infectious disease.

SNEAKY BUGS, SUPERBUGS, AND IMMUNE SUPPRESSION

Disease, Disaster, and Death—a cascading concatenation of calamities.

Death from infectious disease is on the rise. In the sixties and seventies, we thought antibiotics had conquered infectious disease. Then, between 1980 and 1992, deaths from infectious disease increased fifty-eight percent. Because of this surge, infectious diseases have surpassed strokes and accidents as a leading cause of death and now rank behind only heart disease and cancer. Dr. Robert Pinner of the CDC reported this at a meeting of the National Press Club as part of a major news briefing on the threat of emerging diseases. The American Medical Association sponsored the briefing. What is going on here?

One thing that is going on is immune suppression. What happens to an immune system that is confronted with polluted food, air and water, a degraded food supply, the Standard American Diet, the superstition of materialism and ignorance? What happens is that each of these factors impairs immune function. So do the electromagnetic fields that most of us are exposed to every day. The degraded food supply deprives the immune system of micronutrients (vitamins and minerals) that it must have to function at full efficiency. The Standard American Diet, which is a high carbohydrate diet, stimulates the body to produce excess insulin. This causes an overproduction of the kind of eicosanoids (powerful tissue hormones) that, among other mischief, suppress immune function. Superstition and ignorance lead to behaviors and mind-states that create over-stress which causes the over production of adrenal hormones, including cortisol, which suppress immune function. Ignorance and superstition also give rise to depression, as we shall see in a subsequent chapter. Depression depresses immune function right along with mood. People who have studied the immune system consider it a circulating nervous system, because both systems respond to the same neurotransmitters. The neurotransmitters associated with depression depress the immune system. Other neurotransmitters, associated with peace, joy, and love, powerfully strengthen the immune system.

Therefore, you can see that something not so funny happened to many immune systems on the way to the late twentieth century. Meanwhile, what has been going on with the other life forms with which we share Planet Earth? What have the viruses, bacteria, parasites, and yeast been doing? The bacteria and viruses have been busily mutating. Bacteria have had wonderful help from the medical profession in changing themselves into superbugs that are stronger than antibiotics. Few people would now deny that antibiotics in the second half of the twentieth century have been grossly over prescribed. Patients have demanded them and physicians have acquiesced to those demands.

One example is the routine prescription of antibiotics for the common cold. Doctors know that there is no antibiotic that is effective against the virus that causes the common cold. Nevertheless, when a patient comes in with a bad cold and says, "Doc, give me an antibiotic," Doc often does so, or at least did so for many years. The only possible medical justification for that prescription is that it may prevent a secondary infection by bacteria against which the antibiotic is effective. That is like calling down a B-52 strike to carpetbomb the garden because rabbits might get into it. Antibiotics help produce superbugs by killing off all the bacteria except a few that have already mutated to be resistant to the antibiotic. Those bacteria, being the only ones to survive, are able to reproduce themselves in great numbers. Now, the whole bacterial population is resistant to the antibiotic that previously apparently cured the disease. Diseases such as a staphylococcus infection, that previously could easily be cured with an oral antibiotic, now may or may not respond to multiple, simultaneous intravenous antibiotics, which themselves have a serious toxic potential.

While bacteria have had plenty of medical help to change into superbugs, the viruses do not need any help; they just naturally have a talent for mutating. Recent research has shown that some of them mutate best in people who are deficient in selenium. In the US, that is many people. The viruses have taken advantage of this to emerge in new and frightening forms. Some viruses that have been around for a long time are now able, for the first time, to cause disease in human beings. The Ebola virus in Africa and the Hanta virus in the Southwest have recently made headlines.

There are superbugs and there are sneaky bugs. Yeast are sneaky bugs. In small numbers, they are normal inhabitants of the colon. Under the influence of antibiotics, steroids, birth control pills and/or large amounts of alcohol, they increase their numbers to overgrowth proportions. They can live for years in excessive quantities in the human colon without clearly announcing their presence. All the time they are there, however, they are releasing their toxic metabolic products into the blood, over- stressing the immune system and giving rise to a bewildering variety of vague symptoms that were often called neurotic or psychosomatic.

A few years ago, a paper published in the *Journal of the American Medical Association* reported a study of a large number of women with vaginal yeast infections. These researchers found that every time there was a vaginal yeast infection there was also a colon yeast infection. Many doctors must have failed to read that paper, because I see many women who have for years had recurrent vaginal yeast infections. Their infections were treated vaginally without any attention to the colon, which became a reservoir for reinfection of the vagina and gradually undermined immune function.

Parasites are another part of the story. The lab reports that come across my desk in a steady stream tell me that we are in an epidemic of parasitic infections that are generally unsuspected. This is partly because laboratory technicians in the average hospital lab are trained to look for worm eggs in stool specimens, but not to very readily identify other parasites such as *Cryptosporidium* and *Blastocystis*. Fortunately, there is an excellent national reference laboratory, the Great Smokies Medical Laboratory, which does a thorough and reliable job detecting parasites.

Not long ago an eleven-year-old boy was brought in by his parents because he had been diagnosed with Attention Deficit Disorder. He also had episodes of nausea, headache, and a vague, strange, uncomfortable feeling in his abdomen. I thought he probably had a yeast overgrowth and ordered a comprehensive parasitology stool test that is good for detecting yeast. As it turned out, he did not have a yeast overgrowth, but he did have an infection with amoeba. The amoeba responded to treatment. A few months later, in a follow up telephone consultation, the boy's mother told me that he had recently been re-tested at school and no longer had ADD. Headaches, nausea, and abdominal discomfort had also disappeared. This case illustrates the First Tacks Law of Sidney M. Baker, M.D., "When you are sitting on a tack it takes a lot of Ritalin to make it feel good." Many children with an ADD diagnosis would have gotten Ritalin, but this boy was fortunate in having parents that understood the wisdom of finding the cause of the problem rather than masking it with a drug. It takes an awful lot of Ritalin to kill amoebas.

The bottom line is that when a suppressed immune system meets sneaky bugs and superbugs, the result is usually disease, sometimes disaster and, all too often, death. Remember the fifty-eight percent increase in deaths from infectious disease between 1980 and 1992?

Now it is time to consider the two factors that are the root causes of all of the above problems: superstition and ignorance.

SUPERSTITION

Scalding hot water from the shower beat full force on the beautiful upturned face of the young woman whose body lay crumpled in the shower stall. The skin of her face soon began to blister. Large blisters raised, ran together, and burst. Tatters of skin began to spatter the walls of the shower. The hot water supply gave out and still she lay unconscious. Eventually her mother found her there, facial muscles exposed to the now cold water and the skin that had been on her face stuck in shreds on the wall of the shower. Earlier that morning she had taken a dose of opiates, expecting to get a delicious high. After swallowing the tablets, she went to the shower to enjoy the warmth of the water on her skin while the warmth and euphoria of the opiates spread through her consciousness. She miscalculated the dose, however, and as soon as she turned on the hot water, she lost consciousness and slumped into the shower.

Her catastrophic accident was the culmination of a life that she had described as being dedicated to hedonism. She told me that she lived to experience pleasure, the more intense and the more frequent the better. She recognized no value higher than the pleasures of the senses. She had dedicated her considerable talents, beauty, and wealth to the pursuit of pleasure. She had consulted me a couple of years earlier because of depression. I had asked her to consider the possibility that there was more to her reason for being in the world than the pursuit of pleasure. She was willing to consider that and to practice meditation as a way of expanding her consciousness and gaining some awareness of her true purpose in life.

For several months, her depression began to lift and she was hopeful of finding meaning and purpose. Eventually, however, she was not willing to forego the pleasures of marijuana and opiates. While she achieved a measure of peace and well being from meditation, she chose to continue to enjoy the mind—altered states induced by the substances. She believed that she could have the best of both worlds. I told her that I did not believe she could, and that if she continued to abuse drugs, she would stop meditating and experience the inevitable downward spiral to destruction that invariably results from persistent substance abuse. She chose drugs and discontinued her consultations with me. I heard from a mutual friend about her disastrous accident in the shower about a year after I last saw her as a patient.

After sustaining third degree burns over one hundred percent of her face, she was taken to a major teaching hospital where she had numerous operations for skin grafting and restoration of ears, lips, and eye lids that had been completely burned away. The result of months of surgery and suffering was a functional face that was startlingly grotesque. This woman who had been so proud of her beautiful features now had to confront the world with a rigid, grotesque mask of scar tissue. However, she could be glad that her reconstructed lips worked well enough to permit eating and her reconstructed eyelids would cover her corneas enough to prevent their drying and destruction.

She is one of millions of victims of superstition. One definition of superstition is "a belief founded on irrational feelings, especially of fear, and marked by a trust in or reverence for charms, omens, signs, the supernatural, etc." Dr. Chopra has described the prevailing superstition of our culture as, "The superstition of materialism." This is the superstition that only what the five senses, or their technological extensions, can perceive has any reality or value. Material things, then, are the only real and valuable things, the only worthy objects of human endeavor. Such values as love, honor, fidelity, and compassion, not being perceived by the sense of taste, touch, smell, hearing, or sight, are of no value and therefore not worthy of consideration. Faith in this superstition has been a major contributing factor to the pollution, degradation of food supply and abusive lifestyles that we have just been considering. The superstition is the basis of the late twentieth century formula for success: to successfully compete, spy, lie, deceive, and cheat. Several times a year, the media report another fabulously rich individual going to prison as a result of living by this superstition.

Being guided by the superstition of materialism is a virtual, if not absolute, obstacle to experiencing the 100-year healthspan. Fulfillment, peace, and happiness are great allies of the 100-year healthspan. Depression and anxiety are its enemies. Happiness ultimately comes from being in the process of fulfilling one's purpose in life. Taking action every day to fulfill purpose virtually guarantees that some happiness will come into one's life every day. Failure to act to fulfill purpose leads first to anxiety and eventually to depression. Both of these mind-body states produce neurotransmitter and other chemical changes in the body that weaken the immune system, accelerate aging, and substantially shorten the healthspan. When one is in the grips of the superstition of materialism, he cannot even know what his purpose in life is, much less take effective action to fulfill it.

The true purpose in life is always more than the acquisition of material things and the pursuit of pleasure. Purpose in life may include the acquisition and enjoyment of objects but it never stops there. It always includes values that cannot be perceived by any of the senses. Our western civilization has been gripped by this superstition for the past four or five hundred years. For a more thorough and useful discussion of this, see *The Celestine Prophecy*, by James Redfield. We are just beginning to break free of the superstition of materialism, but most people are still trapped in it.

One of the ways in which the superstition of materialism works against the attainment of the 100-year healthspan is by contributing a contemptuous attitude toward the long living. In

Ageless Body, Timeless Mind, Dr. Chopra analyzes the factors contributing to the attainment of 100-year healthspan by many people in Abkhasia. His conclusion was that one of the most powerful supporting factors is the attitude of respect and admiration for the long living. This is due partly to a respect for the wisdom gradually accumulated during a long lifespan. Since wisdom cannot be perceived by the senses, the superstition of materialism considers it worthless and does not see any value to what the long living have gained from experience.

This is not the case in other cultures. In the traditional Cherokee culture, a long living woman was given the title of "War Woman". She sat as a member of the council of elders who made decisions about when and whether the tribe would go to war and what would be done with captives taken in battle. She often had the power of life or death over prisoners of war and indirectly over the men of the tribe, through her influence over whether or not they went into battle.

Once a culture has freed itself from the superstition of materialism, the way is clear for wisdom and those who possess it to be valued and honored. This powerfully supports the 100-year healthspan.

IGNORANCE

"There is only one good, knowledge, and only one evil, ignorance."

—Socrates

A friend used to remark that ignorance is the worst thing in the world. He spoke from his own experience but also on good authority. He was in agreement not only with wise Socrates but also with the wisdom traditions of India, China, and Japan—tradition that goes back five thousand years, as long as there are written records.

The ignorance that is the most dangerous hazard to the 100 year healthspan is ignorance of the answers to the Three Big

Questions: who am I, why am I here, and what is my true relationship to the other people and things in my life? Good and wise people throughout history have devoted their lives to answering the question, "Who am I?" There is the story of a visitor to the monastery where St. Francis of Assisi was living. Deeply moved by the spiritual power and presence of Francis, the visitor went at night to the door of Francis's cell to hear him pray. For hours that night he heard Francis saying, "Who are you, O God, and who am I?"

Of the great religions, Buddhism, and particularly Zen Buddhism, probably has the best developed and most clearly articulated technology for answering the first big question. Zen teachers often lead intensive meditation retreats for their students. The students practice different forms of meditation for as many hours of the twenty-four as they can stay awake. Many people have found satisfying and empowering answers to the questions while attending these retreats. For a clear description of the technology and fascinating accounts of these enlightenment experiences see *The Three Pillars of Zen,* by Phillip Kapleau.

Sometimes, in psychotherapy, I talk with patients about discovering their true selves. It is not unusual for a patient to say, "I don't want to know myself; I might not like me."

I usually say, "I understand that you are afraid, but I absolutely assure you that getting acquainted with yourself will be the most delightful surprise of your life. What you fear you will not like is what people have told you that you are. Everybody who has told you who you are doesn't know you either. In effect, you've been brainwashed with dirty water."

So long as you do not know your true self, or Higher Self, as Chopra puts it, there is always anxiety. As we have noted earlier, anxiety sets off a cascade of biochemical reactions that accelerates the aging process and makes disease more likely.

The second big question is "Why am I here?" When I was the attending psychiatrist on the chemical dependency unit of a psychiatric hospital, I usually asked about purpose in life as part of the evaluation for new patients. About one in fifteen would say that he had no purpose in life, but was alive by chance, or as the result of contraceptive failure. By far the majority knew they had a purpose, but had not a clue about what it was. Most of them said they very much wanted to know. That usually led to a discussion of technologies for finding out and the importance of staying clean and sober. A clear, stabilized, fully alert mind is prerequisite; a mind altered by drugs practically guarantees failure.

Although we have already mentioned the role of failure to fulfill purpose in creating anxiety and depression, this is such an important issue that I would like to develop it further. One of the greatest horrors a person can experience, perhaps the ultimate horror, is to die with the purpose for which one came into life unfulfilled. Everyone knows this on some deep level. To know that the clock is running, life is passing, and purpose is not getting fulfilled is to feel that horror coming closer everyday. The result is a deep anxiety, the source of which is completely unknown to most people, while the experience is all too clear. The anxiety is so painful that many people will go to practically any extreme to dull it. Substance abuse, overwork, and the pursuit of sex, wealth, or power are favorite ways to blunt awareness of this existential anxiety. James Redfield has effectively addressed this issue in *The Tenth Insight*.

If the anxiety goes on too long, it is complicated by despair of ever fulfilling purpose. We believe this despair is the root cause of most, but not all, depression. Since every event in the mind has a corresponding event in the body, this despair gives rise to the imbalances in neurotransmitters, which we know occur in depression. The use of anti-depressant drugs can modulate these transmitter imbalances and give some relief, but they do not bring joy or address the source of the problem. They are also clumsy and imprecise, like doing watch repair with a sledgehammer. It usually happens that as soon as the anti-depressant drug is discontinued, the depression returns. The other side of the coin is that once one knows purpose and takes action every day to fulfill it, happiness comes in to one's life every day. When this happens, your body-mind does its own neurotransmitter balancing and does it precisely and accurately, something no drug can ever do.

This does not mean that there is no stress, pain, or trouble. There is always stress, pain, and trouble associated with human life. What the daily input of happiness means is that there is a counterbalance to the stress, pain and trouble, so that one does not get overwhelmed by them, even in extreme situations such as Nazi concentration camps. For a vivid account of how the discovery and fulfillment of purpose kept a young physician alive through years in Nazi concentration camps see Viktor Frankl's book, *Man's Search for Meaning.*

The last of the three big questions is, who are all these other people in my life, and what is the true nature of my relationship to them? A major factor in the shortening of the healthspan is the stress, conflict and sometimes violence to the point of deadly force, that comes from ignorance of the true nature of the relationship that exists among people. This true nature is that we are so interconnected that it is impossible to do harm to another without also harming one's self or to help another without also helping one's self. The only exception we know to this law is doing harm to another in the fulfillment of one's duty, as when someone uses deadly force that is really necessary and unavoidable in order to protect weak or innocent people.

Ignorance of the inextricable interconnectedness between people leads to people doing harmful things to other people with the expectation that, if they do it cleverly enough, they can avoid bringing harm on themselves. Natural law says otherwise. People do not break natural law; they break themselves upon it. It takes wisdom to see and understand this law because there is often a substantial time lag between hurting another and feeling the resulting damage and pain to one's self. Although the time is often relatively long, it is not long enough to permit the perpetrator to enjoy the 100-year healthspan.

Once this ignorance gives way to knowledge, there is a dramatic shift in one's attitude toward others. "What's in it for me?" gives way to "How can I help? How can I serve?" With this reorientation, much of the stress, conflict, and frustration drains away from relationships and is replaced by peace, love, fulfillment, and happiness. These latter experiences are as strongly supportive of the 100-year healthspan as anger, conflict, frustration, bitterness, and violence are destructive to it.

The last form of ignorance to be mentioned here is unawareness that for maximum probability of attaining the 100-year healthspan, one must not only *know* one's Whole Self, body, mind and spirit, but also *develop and evolve* all three major aspects of that Self simultaneously. This is the second most important discovery that has come from my 40 years of medical practice. We believe it is an essential concept and strategy. Since it appears to be a novel idea, we will develop it in detail in a subsequent chapter, Balancing Whole Self, Strategy.

It is now time to begin to discover the powerful interventions and countermeasures that enable us to meet and overcome these dangerous challenges to possession and enjoyment of our natural birthright.

Often the test of courage is not to die but to live.

—Vittorio Alfieri

Part II:

Knowledge for Claiming Your Birthright

Chapter 3

ATTENTION: POWER FOR YOUR 100-YEAR HEALTHSPAN

A man asked a famous Zen Master, "What is the most important thing in life?"

The Zen Master, who happened to be doing calligraphy, picked up his brush and wrote, "Attention."

The man was puzzled. He said, "I don't understand. Please elaborate."

The Zen Master then wrote, "Attention. Attention."

The man by this time was getting exasperated. In an irritable tone he said, "I don't see anything very subtle or helpful about that. Isn't there anything more you can say?"

The Zen Master then wrote, *"Attention. Attention. Attention."*
—*Anonymous*

In the preceding chapter, you read about a daunting array of obstacles and hazards to claiming your birthright from nature. To overcome these obstacles you need skill, will and power. This book is a major resource for learning the skills. You can supply the will by tapping into the invincible evolutionary thrust of nature. In Chapter 5, "Strengthening The Power of Attention", we tell you how to do that. The third vital ingredient is power. The dictionary defines power as the ability to act. In this case, power means the ability to act by using the skills that you are about to learn, as well as some you already know. There is abundant power available to you, but you must unlock it before you can use it. It is like standing beside a BMW. The vehicle has the power to take you wherever roads run; but if you do not have the key that opens the door and operates the ignition, that power is not doing you any good. Attention is your key to unlocking the power to claim your birthright. Attention is defined as *the concentrated direction of mental powers, the power of the faculty of mental concentration.* When you concentrate and direct your mental powers onto the skills you are about to learn, you unlock and gain access to all the power you need to apply these skills to claim your birthright.

FIRST ENCOUNTER

"...Ye spread and span like the catholic man who hath mightily won

God out of knowledge and good out of infinite pain

And sight out of blindness and purity out of a stain."
— Sidney Lanier, in "The Marshes of Glynn"

My first encounter with the power of attention was not the result of lofty spiritual or scientific investigation. Terror and horror drove me to it. One spring morning in 1975, I arrived at my office early, before anyone else. When I looked at my appointment book, I was stunned. The page was blank! There were no patients scheduled. Fourteen years earlier, I had begun practice as the first psychiatrist in southwest Georgia. From the beginning, I had a large, busy practice—too busy, in fact. I lived what Bob Dylan sang: "All of us at times may work too hard, to get it too fast and too much, and everyone can fill his life up with things he can see, but he just cannot touch."

I had chosen to let greed drive my life too far out of balance—too much contact with the raw, bleeding edges of emotional suffering of my patients, not enough time to deal with my own suffering and need for healing. My own emotional pain had become severe. I chose to numb it with alcohol. During a disastrous decade of abusing alcohol, I alienated most of my referral sources and did my reputation grievous harm. I knew too well what the poet Omar Khayyam meant when he wrote, "Indeed the Idols I have loved so long have done my credit in the eyes of men much wrong! Have drowned my honor in a shallow cup and sold my reputation for a song."

I had known that my practice was dwindling, but as long as I was seeing two or three patients a day, I could maintain denial that there was a serious problem. *No* patients, however, was a reality check! The reality that I saw clearly written on that blank page of the appointment book was the prophecy of my ruin. Without patients, I would be unable to support my family. I would be forced into bankruptcy and humiliation. The people I had failed would abandon me. Not only was I facing what appeared to me the ultimate horror, but also I had to face it alone, because I had alienated most of my friends. My humiliated ego would not permit me to turn to family members and those few remaining friends who could have supported me in this crisis. I felt totally isolated and abandoned.

I felt suffocated and increasingly weak as I stood in my consulting room. Suddenly too feeble to remain standing, I collapsed into a recliner beside my desk, pushed it back and lay there in utter devastation, helplessness, hopelessness and horror. Out of sheer desperation, without any thought of why or how, I began to visualize myself as a tiny speck floating in an infinite universe of love.

As I focused my attention on this vision, something absolutely magical and unexpected began to happen. The horror, terror, shame, guilt, and suffocation that had been consuming me began to dissolve into a profound experience of peace and love! Not only was there peace and love where there had moments before been horror and terror, but there was also the experience of awe and wonder, as a whole new universe began to open to me. It was a universe of light, peace, unlimited freedom, and unconditional love. It was as though I had walked through a looking glass and in a moment had passed from hell into heaven. I felt like the cowboy who rode his horse to the rim of the Grand Canyon, looked in, and exclaimed, "Wow! Something sure happened!"

I have been using the power of attention to explore this Grand Canyon of higher awareness ever since. The discoveries become more exciting and the unfolding vistas more magnificent all the time. On that spring morning, with the horror and suffocation of a few minutes before transmuted into an experience of peace, love and wonder, I set out to explore this new dimension of awareness which I called "the non-physical universe." I discovered that I could enter this level of awareness, this dimension of reality, at will by focusing my attention on the visual image that had opened it to me initially. Once in this awareness, I could explore it as much as I wished by keeping attention focused on whatever was unfolding at the time. Then, when issues in the space-time dimension of reality, the ordinary waking level of awareness, needed attention, I could switch back into space-time by focusing attention on whatever needed to be dealt with.

This exploration of the non-physical universe was a totally different experience from daydreaming. I know; I have done much of both. During my solitary boyhood, I spent hours each day in fantasy. I well remember how that felt: interesting at first, but then disappointing, boring, insipid and eventually, unpleasant, constricting, and agitating. In those fantasies, I always created the story and wrote the script. Now, when my attention was on the non-physical universe, I was not creating; I was observing. It was like being on a float trip, enjoying the ever-changing scene that unfolded as the canoe rounded each bend in the river. What I was observing in the non-physical universe was definitely not created by the intellect that created my boyhood and adult fantasies. The effect was different, too. I never tired of exploring the non-physical universe. It was always nourishing, energizing, and clarifying. Then, when I came back to deal with the issues in space-time dimension (seeing a patient, playing with the children, enjoying gardening with Genevieve, running errands), I was able to use the enhanced energy and clarity to function better than I had before.

I cannot imagine a more powerful initiation into the power of attention. In those transforming moments in my empty consulting room one spring morning in 1975, nothing in the physical universe had changed. My appointment book was just as blank after I passed through the looking glass from hell into heaven as it had been before. No patient had come to sit in my waiting room. My cash flow had not increased one dime. The only change had been a change in my awareness—and in my freedom. I was no longer trapped in the space-time dimension of reality. Although nothing in there had changed, the change in my awareness preceded a major constructive change in my physical world. No longer paralyzed by fear and shame, I was able to do what was necessary to begin to repair the damage I had done.

Patients gradually returned and I was able to cultivate new referral sources. My practice revived. Not only did it revive, but also I was able to be of far more help to my patients. My transforming experience with the power of attention changed my life forever in a radically favorable way. It opened the possibility for this book. It also immediately empowered me to be with and to guide many patients who were as desperate as I had been. Out of my own experience in a time of extreme crisis and desperate need, I was able as never before to assist them in their discovery of a new level of awareness, which they had to experience in order to solve their own massive problems. Now that I knew how to use the power of attention to access a higher level of awareness and thinking, I could teach and lead others to use this method to solve their own problems. This ability has been useful countless times, but never more so than when I was treating prisoners from the local jails.

Before the great flood of 1994, I was working part time in the local mental health center, where I masterminded jailbreaks for convicted drug dealers. That was not my job description. My job was to treat prisoners who were brought in from the local jails. Most of them had been convicted of dealing drugs and had been in jail for months awaiting transfer to various prisons, where they would serve long sentences. Not surprisingly, most of them were anxious and seriously depressed. In those circumstances, not to be anxious and seriously depressed would require that they be psychotic or very highly spiritually developed. The ones I saw gave no evidence of either condition.

The constraints of the mental health center limited me to spending ten or fifteen minutes with each prisoner and prescribing the oldest, cheapest anti-depressant drugs. Trying to help those prisoners within those constraints was like trying to stop a charging rhinoceros with a B.B. gun and a fly swatter. Clearly, I had to have something more. Here was a job for the power of attention! However, how to help these people, who had not spent years studying metaphysics, to turn on that power was a difficult question.

Wayne Dyer to the rescue with *Real Magic!*

Dr. Wayne Dyer has written the best introduction I have ever seen to discovering and turning on the power of attention. He named the book *Real Magic*. So many of my private patients had made such good use of that knowledge that I bought a supply of the paperback edition and kept the books in my desk at the mental health center.

When I saw a patient who looked ready; i.e., desperate enough to try almost anything, I would go into my *Real Magic* spiel. I said, "It doesn't look as though you're going to be able to get your body out of jail right now, but would you be interested in getting your mind out?" At that point, the prospect of getting anything of his out of jail was attractive to the prisoner. I had his attention. I would then reach into the desk, pull out a copy of *Real Magic*, hold it where he could see it and say, "In this book there are detailed instructions about how you can get your mind out of jail." Then I would hand the book to the prisoner. He would look skeptical, puzzled, and hopeful at the same time, and leave carrying the book in one of his manacled hands.

It usually happened that the next time I saw him he would not look quite so depressed. We would then discuss the principles Dyer set forth in the book, including discovery of purpose and using the power of attention.

I remember one prisoner, who had been severely depressed, coming back for a follow up visit looking happy. He had been studying and applying the Real Magic principles of being on purpose and mentally sending love to other people. These actions required him to focus his attention in a way he had never done before. I asked him if he had learned to get his mind out of jail. He said that he had. I asked, "If you had the choice of getting your mind out of jail and leaving your body in or getting your body out and leaving your mind in, which would you choose?"

Without a moment's hesitation he replied, "I would get my mind out and leave my body in."

Another prisoner, whom I will call Jim, was in jail on suspicion of arson. He was confined in a cell with a teenage gang member who fancied himself very tough and acted psychotic. For long intervals each day, he beat on the bars of his cell with his metal drinking cup and screamed. He also looked as though he might, at any moment, attack Jim.

Jim found this combination of clamor and menace nerve wracking, to say the least. I had given him a copy of *Real Magic*, which he was studying with intensity born of desperation. After reading about the power of unconditional love, he began to mentally send it to his cellmate. Within forty-eight hours, his cellmate's attitude had radically changed. The young gang member began bringing Jim his food tray when it was pushed under the door. He said to Jim, "I'm not going to scream anymore or beat on the door except when you are out of the cell." He was as good as his word. One day he wrapped himself in toilet paper and set it on fire, but he did it when Jim was not in the cell.

With this combination of the power of attention and the truth in *Real Magic*, I was able to help quite a few desperate prisoners to mentally escape from a prison that had confined them long before they landed in the Dougherty County jail. You will find the story of a spectacular mental and spiritual jailbreak in the chapter, "Why Am I Here?"

HISTORICAL PERSPECTIVES

These experiences with the power of attention, although impressive to me, were hardly new discoveries. Writings about the power of attention go back as far as written history and the knowledge probably much farther. In the Jewish and Christian traditions, God spoke the universe into being. Before the word had to come the thought. Before the thought there had to be consciousness, and for consciousness to result in a thought, there had to be attention, the concentrated direction of mental powers. In the book of Proverbs, there is the statement, "As a man thinketh in his heart so is he." In the New Testament, according to the Gospel of St. John, "The word was made flesh." The Greek that is translated "word" in John's Gospel is *logos*, which entails much more than thought or spoken words. Most scholars say that it means all knowledge. For there to be the word, there had first to be thought; and for the thought to occur there had to be the focus of attention in consciousness.

In the Buddhist tradition, the *Dhamma Pada* is a record of the sayings of the Buddha. The first chapter begins with the statement that we are what we think. It goes on the say that with our thoughts we make the world. Not only that, but if we speak or act with an impure mind, trouble will follow us as the wheel follows the ox that draws the cart. On the other hand, if we speak or act with a pure mind, happiness will follow us like our shadow.

If you prefer being followed by happiness rather than trouble, you may feel an interest in what it means to speak and act with a pure rather than an impure mind. This we will discuss in detail in the two chapters on "Balancing Whole Self." By way of preview, a pure mind refers to a level of awareness that is called "The Field of Pure Consciousness," or "The Unified Field." This level of consciousness, which is higher than ordinary waking consciousness, develops when the attention is focused in a way that frees awareness from the limitations of emotion, intellect, and ego.

Many modern authors have written about the power of attention. In the last century, James Allen wrote *As A Man Thinketh.* This little book is well worth reading for an understanding of how awareness of the power of attention had evolved at the time of the nineteenth century. Among contemporary authors, Dyer, in *Real Magic,* has written what we believe is the best introduction to an understanding of the power of attention. Deepak Chopra, M.D. has made a major contribution to this knowledge with many of his books, beginning with *Quantum Healing* and, more recently, *The Return of Merlin* and *The Way of the Wizard.* His audiocassette album, *The Higher Self,* speaks eloquently and powerfully to this issue. James Redfield in *The Celestine Prophecy, The Tenth Insight,* and their accompanying experiential guides has shown how the power of attention is driving a rapid and radical expansion of consciousness in our whole culture. His writings offer practical, systematic instructions on how to focus attention to enrich daily life, accelerate personal spiritual evolution, and more completely fulfill one's personal mission. These authors and teachers are at the forefront of a growing group who are contributing to an increasing cultural awareness that attention is supremely powerful, if we but know how to use it.

HOW IT WORKS

We do not yet know everything about how attention works to exert the power of life and death, health and disease, happiness and misery, but we know a great deal. For five thousand years, Vedic seers and other enlightened individuals have known and written that the whole flow of the universe is from consciousness to matter. "With our thoughts we make the world."

In the last decade, Dr. Candace Pert, at the National Institutes of Health, has clearly demonstrated that the flow is from mind to molecules. She deserves a Nobel Prize for finally proving that thought and emotion precede molecules, and not vice versa. The debate about that had gone on for a long time. She also demonstrated that every thought and every emotion has its signature pattern of messenger molecules: neurotransmitters, endorphins, and hormones.

Others have made important contributions as well. Chopra has observed that when you think, you are practicing brain chemistry. Redfield wrote, "Where attention goes, energy flows." Once you understand this concept, you are beginning to understand the mechanics of the power of attention. Dyer teaches that what you put your attention on expands in your life. When you apply the Redfield principle, this is easy to understand. What you put your attention on gets increased energy, so it is natural for it to grow stronger and expand. What you take your attention away from has its energy input reduced, so it has to weaken or wither away.

The man with a heart attack phobia keeps fearful attention on something going terribly wrong with his heart. This increases the probability of the event that he fears. Were he to re-direct his attention to fulfilling his purpose in life, fulfillment and happiness would grow stronger. The phobia, deprived of energy, would wither away. His heart could then breathe a sigh of relief and pump away happily.

Dyer has pointed out that the only thing over which we have full control in this life is our thoughts. If we can have control over only one thing, thoughts are that thing, because "With our thoughts we make the world." Since we control thought through the process of attention, it becomes clear what power attention potentially has. By focusing your attention on what you want to have growing larger in your life and taking your attention away from what you want to have disappear from your life, you take charge of your destiny and the direction of your life in a fundamentally powerful way.

Measurement Theory

The branch of modern physics called Measurement Theory has systematically studied the interaction between attention and material things. The basic principle of Measurement Theory is, "The attention of the observer does something to the object of observation." What a remarkable statement! Attention, a very non-physical thing, has an influence on a material object!

I had a conversation with Dr. Roy Curtain, a brilliant physicist who has invented a powerful electrodiagnostic instrument called the Interro. Roy told me about an experience he had while on contract with the Department of Defense during the Cold War. His contract called for him to determine to what degree strategic military planners in the Pentagon could mentally access the thoughts of military planners in the Kremlin. The Cold War was threatening to turn hot, so this was an important national security issue. As part of this project, Roy programmed a computer to be a random number generator. After satisfying himself that the system was working as programmed, he called several colleagues into the computer room, where he asked them focus their attention on a particular number. As they did so, the computer, which was programmed to produce numbers at random, began to generate that particular number with a greater frequency than any other. The increased frequency was statistically significant. Eventually, the computer reverted to its program, but there was an interval during which the attention of those observers had a measurable, statistically significant influence on the object, the computer.

Not being satisfied with this experiment (computers seem almost capable of intelligent thought), Roy devised a more purely mechanical machine. It was a device like a large pinball machine, with a compartment at the upper end containing many steel balls. Below this compartment, there were a number of baffles positioned to direct an equal number of steel balls into each of four compartments at the bottom of the device. After calibrating the machine to function as designed, Roy called his colleagues in again. They all put their attention on the same lower compartment. When the balls were released, sure enough, more of them collected in the compartment that was receiving the attention of the observers.

In case you are wondering, Roy determined that strategic planners in the Pentagon indeed could access the thoughts in the minds of strategic planners in the Kremlin. He also discovered that strategic planners in the Kremlin were more skilled at accessing the thoughts of strategic planners in the Pentagon than vice versa. Fortunate indeed that the Cold War ended before it turned hot. Since Dr. Curtain's experiments, other researchers have repeatedly shown that the output of random systems responds to individual attention.

Now there is further evidence that random systems also respond to collective attention. A working paper from the Princeton Engineering Anomalies Research Lab (PEAR), School of Engineering/Applied Science, Princeton University, describes an experiment in which researchers put a random event generator in ten organized group environments. The participants in the groups paid no attention to the random event generator (REG). Their attention was on the topic of the meeting. Nevertheless, the REG showed highly significant deviations in output while the groups were in session. The ten sessions included six research conferences, two ritual religious events, a business meeting, and a group field investigation of an environmental anomaly. The REG emitted the most unusual pattern of activity during periods described as high in group attention, cohesiveness and shared emotion.

So the information continues to come in, this time from a laboratory in a prestigious Eastern university, that the power of attention is a far more potent force for creating events in the material world than a culture trapped in the superstition of materialism had ever been imagined.

The Maharishi Effect

We have just considered two examples of scientific evidence that the power of the mind can affect machines. These experiments lend support to the concept of a "consciousness field," which is a group-driven force, proposed by Rupert Sheldrake and others. Evidence that this "consciousness field" can also influence large social organizations was published more than ten years ago in *The Journal of Conflict Resolution* and *The Journal of Mind and Behavior*. Long before that, it was known that the consciousness field created by an angry mob resulted in some individuals doing horribly destructive things that they would never consider doing alone. *People of the Lie*, by Scott Peck, M.D., is an exposition of this. A different kind of consciousness field, called a "coherent consciousness field," can have the opposite effect. It can cause behavior that is more loving and evolutionary than the individual would ordinarily consider.

This new evidence was discovered in the '70's when Transcendental Meditation (TM) was a fad and millions of people were doing it. TM is known to create consciousness that is more coherent (clear, focused, harmonious, and integrated) than ordinary waking consciousness. During coherent consciousness, brain waves also become more coherent, as measured by an electroencephalograph (EEG).

People began to notice that, in cities where there were large numbers of people doing TM, crime rates fell and economic conditions improved. This became remarkable enough that the sociologists devised an experiment to see if there was a causal relationship between a large number of people meditating in an area and improved quality of life for everyone. Perhaps this was just a random occurrence that could be explained by chance.

Several cities were selected for their large number of meditators. Control cities were selected where there were not many meditators. Other characteristics, such as population, type of industry, climate, and political system were similar. The study was conducted for three years. It showed that in the cities where at least one percent of the population was regularly doing TM, or a fraction of one percent was regularly doing an advanced TM technique called the TM Sidhi Program, there was a one to two percent per year decrease in violent crime. During the same period, violent crime increased in the control cities. Statistical analysis indicated that there were fewer than five chances in 100 that this would happen by chance.

In Washington, D.C., in 1981 and 1982, when there were the specified number of meditators active in the city, there was a 10% decrease in violent crime each year. Then the number of meditators fell below the critical threshold. The rest is sad history.

The most spectacular example of the effect of a sufficient number of people creating a coherent consciousness field was reported in *The Journal of Conflict Resolution*. For two weeks in September 1993, at the height of the Lebanese war, forty thousand TM meditators went to the area around Lebanon and did TM. 197 meditators who did the TM Sidhi Program joined them. During those two weeks war deaths decreased more than 75%, from forty per day to ten per day. There was also a reduction in property destruction and crime. When the numbers were crunched for statistical significance, the result was the most highly statistically significant event ever analyzed. When the meditators went home after two weeks, death, crime, and destruction from the war returned to previous levels. This discovery was named the Maharishi Effect in honor of the founder of the TM movement.

It seems incredible that such spectacularly favorable results from the use of the power of attention would be ignored for over a decade. These reports were published in respected, peer reviewed scientific journals. The only way we can account for this astonishing oversight is that most people were not at a level of consciousness necessary to understand the significance of what was reported. They were unable to see the potential for revolutionizing the quality of life for whole countries and, in fact, the world. We believe that many people who read this book will be at a level of consciousness that will enable them to understand and see the potential.

The take-away from this chapter is that the most wonderful thing you can do for yourself and the world is to focus your attention in such a way that your awareness expands and your energy field becomes more coherent. Then you can recruit others to make similar use of the power of attention, and to encourage still others to do so until the critical threshold of one percent of the population of your region is reached and the quality of life of everyone pulls up to a higher level. After reading this, if you are not already using the power of attention in this way, we hope you will be inspired to pay close attention to the instructions in Chapter 5 on how to do so. Having learned how, we encourage you to put those instructions to practical use immediately. If you are already using attention in this way, I hope you will feel inspired to give more time and more energy to this fundamentally vital practice for the achievement of the 100-year healthspan for yourself and many other people.

PLACEBO AND NOCEBO

Another fascinating manifestation of the power of attention is the placebo effect. Wise physicians know that the patient's belief system has a powerful influence on the outcome of an illness. Substances the physician believes are completely inert, such as starch, can have a strong beneficial effect if the patient is convinced it is beneficial. It can even have a beneficial effect on several different and unrelated conditions.

A dramatic example of the placebo effect is a surgical procedure called the "internal mammary ligation". A number of years ago, when surgical intervention for coronary insufficiency and angina was just beginning, a surgeon decided that it might be possible to get more blood to flow through constricted coronary arteries if an artery indirectly connected to them was tied off. This is called the internal mammary artery. He began to do the procedure on an experimental basis. To his delight, most of the patients received dramatic relief from angina. He published his findings. Other physicians replicated them. Soon, internal mammary ligation was the most popular surgical procedure performed by cardiovascular surgeons.

In the field of medicine, there are always skeptics and naysayers. Sure enough, one of these decided that there was no way tying off the internal mammary artery could increase blood flow to the heart. He devised an experiment in which coronary artery patients were randomly assigned to one of two groups. One group got the procedure described above. The other group received a sham procedure. The skin was opened and then sewed up again, without anything being done to the internal mammary artery. None of the patients knew who had the sham procedure and who had the actual operation. The physicians who evaluated the results of the two procedures did not know which was which. This is the famous double blind, placebo controlled scientific study that is the gold standard for scientific proof in medicine. When the experiment was completed and the results were analyzed, it was discovered that both groups received marked benefit. Moreover, there was no difference in the benefit to the patients who had the real procedure and those who had the sham procedure!

Our understanding of this remarkable result is that both the actual and the sham operations focused the patients' attention strongly and dramatically on the expectation of recovery. Since, as we have seen, the attention of the observer has an effect on a machine, it does not seem surprising that the attention of the observer on his own body would have an effect. When the attention is on the expectation of benefit or cure, that is the effect that is likely to actually occur. Do you feel a growing appreciation for the power of attention?

The placebo effect has a long and distinguished history in the art and science of medical practice. Until the second half of the twentieth century, physicians knew and valued it as a major therapeutic modality. Throughout most of the history of medical practice, there have not been effective drugs or surgical procedures. Practitioners and patients had to depend on the power of attention, and the power of attention manifests partly as the placebo effect. When the country doctor was called to see a patient who was seriously ill, he usually had no effective drug to assist the patient's recovery. He would sometimes manufacture "medicine" by rolling pills from bread. These would be presented to the patient as a potent remedy. With attention focused on the object, and therefore on the expectation for recovery, the patient would swallow the bread pills and recovery would often be accelerated.

Another way the placebo effect could be triggered was to give the patient a favorable prognosis although the actual prognosis was grave. Again, attention was focused on the expectation of recovery. The attention of the observer (the patient's mind), did something to the object (the patient's body). The converse is true as well; giving a patient a negative prognosis can be devastating to both the patient and his/her family. Studies have shown that families much prefer to be given overly rosy prognoses.

Recent scientific research has given us at least a partial explanation of what the attention of the observer does to the object, in this case the body-mind. Pert, as previously noted, has demonstrated that every thought and every feeling has its signature of neurochemicals and hormones that powerfully influence physiology. When thoughts are of recovery and mood is hopeful, the body produces neurochemicals, including endorphins, neurotransmitters and hormones, that actually support recovery. When thoughts are of decline and death, mood is depressed. Then, other hormones and neurotransmitters are produced that contribute to the expected outcome.

This gives rise to what Bernie Siegel, M.D., has called the "nocebo effect". Oncologists and others may induce the nocebo effect by telling the patient that there is no hope for him and approximately when he will die of cancer. The patient then produces the neurochemicals and hormones that support fulfillment of the prophecy of death.

You may remember that Ken, whose case I briefly presented in Chapter 1, had been given a death sentence to be executed in four months. He chose not to accept the death sentence and the nocebo effect for several reasons. The most fundamental was probably his strong will to live. He had spent his life overcoming large and difficult obstacles, so when presented with this death sentence, he treated it as just another obstacle to be overcome. Another factor was his strong relationship with his daughter, who knew from her own experience the great self-healing power of the body-mind. Perhaps part of Ken's rejection of the nocebo effect and his subsequent recovery was my clear, emphatic statement to him at the first visit. I told him that I believed he could recover, that he did not have to die that December, and that if he could fully activate his self-healing powers he probably would recover.

We wonder why inducing the nocebo effect has become so popular in conventional medicine. Perhaps it is because conventional medicine has made a fetish of being scientific, to the point of disdain for the age-old art of medical practice. Science depends on statistics, and statistics about life and death are easily calculated. Essentially, what the oncologists and other physicians who deal with deadly diseases cite to the patient are the statistics about what happens to most people who have this disease or condition. This unfortunate approach ignores the power of the self-healing mechanism of the body-mind and the uniqueness of each individual. Even the most conventional physician knows that there is occasionally someone who defies the statistics and recovers from an illness that is statistically 100% fatal. Most conventional physicians, however, find this offensive to their belief system, so they ignore it.

Many AIDS patients have proved the power of the placebo response; their positive outlook and disbelief of the nature of their disease has resulted in long lives without clinical disease, even though the virus was still there.

Another factor opposing the use of the placebo response in conventional medicine is a phobia of inducing "false hope." There seems to be a belief that despair is true and hope is false. Siegel has compellingly argued that there is no such thing as false hope, because so long as there is hope, there is a chance that the attention of the observer will do something so favorable to the object that the hope will be fulfilled. Conventional physicians will often say at some point in treating a disease that is considered incurable, "There is nothing more that I can do." Dr. Siegel contends that there is always something more the physician can do. It may be to prescribe medications that ease pain and make the patient's life more comfortable, to pray with the patient, or listen to him. For any physician who understands the power of attention, these are recognized and valued as powerful therapies.

Here is another example of the placebo effect. During the years we lived in Albany, Georgia, a local healer cured cancer with grape juice. From time to time, he would give his protocol for the cancer cure in the letters to the editor section in *The Albany Herald*. His patients published testimonials of cures in the same column. Apparently, several of his patients went into long remissions. If the cancer cure would work when administered by Mr. Wortman, why could physicians not get it to work?

Over forty years of medical practice have led me to believe that healing is a multi-dimensional process. I think that I can identify several of these dimensions. The first is the placebo response. The second is the biochemical and structural change, if any, caused by the treatment. If a patient takes thyroid hormone when she is deficient in that substance, biochemical changes take place. When an orthopedic surgeon reduces an open fracture or replaces a diseased hip joint, structural change takes place. This is another dimension of healing.

A third dimension, we believe, is the transfer of energy from the healer to the patient. Robert Becker, M.D., author of *The Body Electric*, contends that we are energy beings before we are physical beings. Just as we have a physical body, we also have an energy body, which structures and controls the physical body. The best, and probably the only, way to change an energy field is with another energy field. By definition, an energy field is a localized concentration of energy that has the ability to influence other energy fields.

The most powerful energy we know is called love. The most powerful healers are those who feel powerful love. As Willa Cather said in *A Course in Miracles*, "Where there is great love there are always miracles." We have seen many healers. All of them have been extraordinarily loving people. We have never seen a hateful healer. For healing to take place on this dimension, the energy of love must be transmitted from the healer to the patient. The most powerful healers know how to do this with their minds. The effect can often be intensified through touch. There are healers who transmit healing energy through the laying on of hands. The therapeutic touch technique of Dr. Delores Krieger and the healing technique called Reiki are examples.

The giving of substance is another way of transmitting energy. When our country doctor was rolling the bread pills to give to the patient for whom there was no known active medicine, he transmitted some of his love for the patient to the pills. When the patient swallowed the pills, he swallowed a dose of that healing energy along with the bread. The process of handing the pills to the patient also communicated healing energy. If the physician, or other healer, loves the treatment as well as the patient, the benefits are amplified.

There is one other crucially important consideration in this dimension of healing. For this transfer of healing energy to take place, the healer must transmit it, but transmission alone is not enough. For the process to work, the patient must receive what is transmitted. We may be less than a mile from a radio transmitter that is operating at 50,000 watts. We may have a radio turned on, but if it is tuned to a different frequency from that of the transmitter, we will not get the signal. A healer may have the ability to transmit powerful energy; but if the patient is not attuned to receiving it, the healing process will not occur, or will be much less than it could be. Attention largely determines the attunement of the individual. Remember, "As you think so shall you be."

If the patient comes to the encounter with the healer with the expectation of benefit, and attention is focused on the thought, "This experience is going to benefit me," the patient's mind is likely to be tuned to the same frequency as the healer's mind; effective transmission of healing energy will probably occur. If the patient goes into the healing encounter with his attention on the idea, "I *know* that this is going to benefit me," the patient's mind and the healer's mind are likely to lock onto the same frequency. Then healing is highly probable. If you want to benefit from an encounter with a healer, go to the encounter with your attention focused on the expectation and intention of experiencing healing. If you want to be virtually assured of healing, go in to the encounter *knowing* that you will be healed.

How to focus attention effectively is obviously a crucially important subject. We will tell you how in Chapter 5. In later chapters, we will consider how to focus attention on the healing energy of love. A crucial part of this process is to find your answers to The Big Questions: Who am I? Why am I here? What is my relationship to the other people and things in my life?

As I wrote in the previous chapter, I believe that the root cause of sickness, suffering, and disorder is ignorance. The most devastating ignorance is ignorance of one's true nature as a human being. Almost as dangerous is ignorance of one's purpose in life and of the true nature of the relationship between one's self and others. The use of focused attention is the most reliable way to free oneself from this ignorance by attaining appropriate knowledge and wisdom. The technology of using focused attention to accomplish these crucially important achievements will be the subject of chapters six through ten.

Although we consider attention primary in claiming and enjoying your birthright from nature, it is certainly not the only way. In order to claim your birthright as swiftly and surely as possible and enjoy it to the fullest, it is also necessary to create balance and harmony on the physical and mental levels. I will discuss this in detail in the chapters on energy and biochemistry and in Part III.

Conviction is worthless unless it is converted into conduct.

—Thomas Carlyle

Chapter 4

APPLYING the POWER of ATTENTION

INTRODUCTION

Since the power of attention is the power for the 100-year healthspan, there are many ways that it can be applied. In this chapter we give examples of its application to such diverse aspects of life as crisis management, strengthening and using intuition, increasing synchronicities, healing emotional disorders, and creating the very basis of health.

ATTENTION AND CRISIS MANAGEMENT

Balanced consciousness is of incalculable value in day to day life. It is of even greater value during a crisis. After I had been doing zazen (Zen meditation) for about a year, I decided to have a hernia repair. It was my first major surgical operation. I was surprised at the calmness I felt while driving to the hospital for the procedure. I took my zazen mat and round sitting cushion into the hospital room. That night, I sat on the mat and cushion facing the wall in the hospital room and did my usual meditation. After I had meditated for a few minutes, I heard the door open. There was a long silence, then a nurse asked, "Are you all right?"

"Yes, thank you," I answered, without moving. After another minute or two, I heard the door close. I was up again the next morning to meditate before it was time to take the pre-op medication. I went to surgery feeling extraordinarily calm and peaceful. After surgery, I never took any medicine for pain. Without the balancing of awareness that came from meditation, the experience would have been more frightening and painful.

There have been other times when meditation and the experience of pure consciousness were of extraordinary help. The most extreme example was what happened during the ten days when Andy was dying. During those days I alternated among standing by Andy's bed, searching feverishly through the medical school's library to gather enough references to persuade Andy's attending physician to give him the intravenous vitamin C that I knew would provide the best chance of surviving *Pneumocystis* pneumonia, walking in a nearby park, and meditating my way into the field of pure consciousness. Pure consciousness is a great place to visit when things are going terribly wrong in space/time. It is a great place because, in the field of pure consciousness, nothing ever goes wrong: one of the qualities of the field is perfect orderliness. Spending an hour a day in that field where everything is always peaceful and absolutely perfect provided the balance that we had to have in order to deal with the most wrenching and devastating crisis of our lives, and deal with it far better than we could have possibly done otherwise.

Things were truly terrible in the space/time dimension of reality. Andy was suffering and dying. We were suffering and grieving. His attending physicians were sneering at my pleas to use enough vitamin C to improve his chances of survival. One day, while other family members were standing by Andy's bed, Genevieve and I were resuscitating ourselves from the suffocating atmosphere of the intensive care unit by walking in the park. While I was walking and feeling the horror of watching Andy slowly die, I recalled something I had read long ago. It had been written by a man who was intimately acquainted with the dimension beyond space-time, which can be reached through the power of attention. I spoke his words to Genevieve: "And all will be well, and all will be well, and all will be well, and all will be very, very well."

Genevieve squeezed my hand and said, "Yes, I know that."

Neither one of us would have known that had we not regularly been visiting the field of pure consciousness, where all was already very, very well. Those regular visits, far more than the welcome walks in the park, enabled us to maintain our balance during a time of extreme stress.

There are two important things to know about using balanced awareness to enhance your functioning, your skillful crisis management—and sometimes your survival. First, the time to secure your access to the field of pure consciousness is when the stress level is relatively low, not when you are going through a crisis. The best time to do it is when things are running relatively smoothly in your life. Securing your connection and access to the Field is challenging enough, as we hope you are about to discover. You still might be driven to it in a crisis, as I was in the spring of 1975, but that is not a smart bet. Most people are driven to other less favorable responses.

If you start now and steadily build your power to access pure consciousness, you will be like the man in the parable in the New Testament who built his house on a rock. When the flood and the storms came, although they beat on the house, they could not destroy it.

The other thing to know is that when you need meditation most you are least likely to do it. In times of stress and crisis most people think, "I don't have time to meditate", so they do not—and deprive themselves of the power and clarity to seize the opportunities and avoid the dangers in the crisis. Martin Luther's biographer quoted him as saying, "I have so much to do today that I'm going to have to spend an extra hour on my knees."

Gerald Jampolski's advice is, "Give to your meditation the same priority you would give to an attack of diarrhea."

If you heed the words of these wise men you will never regret it, and you will always be glad that you did.

ATTENTION AND THE POWER OF INTUITION

There is another application of attention that is crucial to attainment of the 100-year healthspan: paying attention to intuition. Intuition is defined as a direct knowledge or awareness of something, without conscious reasoning or intellectual activity. Although disdained by science, some of the most important scientific discoveries, such as the Theory of Relativity, were made using intuition, and then validated by the scientific method. Here are some examples of the value of paying attention to intuition and the hazards of ignoring it.

I finished reading a short section in *The Wheel of Death,* by Zen Master Philip Kapleau. I laid the book on the family room table and stood up. At that moment, Genevieve walked into the room and said in a strange voice, "Ricky is dead. Someone just phoned to say he killed himself early this morning."

I felt a wave of gooseflesh start at the base of my neck and spread upward over the scalp and downward to my thighs. Ricky was a close friend of our seventeen-year old son. He had been almost like an adopted son to us. He had accompanied us many times on our weekends at our cabin on the Alapaha River. We knew that for months Ricky had been torn between the drug-culture lifestyle of most of his friends and the different lifestyle of the Woodard family. Lately he had been spending more time with his druggy friends. We later heard that, immediately before shooting himself, he had been using drugs and had wrecked his van not far from his house. Thinking that he had killed the other occupants of the van, he walked home, picked up a pistol and shot himself in the head.

My goose-flesh was caused by a feeling of horror at Ricky's suicide, but even more by sudden awe and understanding of a strange compulsion I had felt for the past six weeks to memorize the memorial service from *The Wheel of Death.* About six weeks earlier, I had been at the Rochester Zen Center where Roshi Kapleau was the Abbot. After attending a meditation retreat, I bought the book. I found the knowledge so powerful that I ran a fever for hours after reading it, and had trouble sleeping that night. From the time that I read the book until the morning we learned of Ricky's death, I had felt compelled to memorize the entire memorial service. After meditation each morning, I learned a segment of it. Just before Genevieve walked into the room, I had finished committing to memory the last segment, and had recited the entire service from memory. I had not understood the urgency of the intuition that I should do this until the moment Genevieve brought news of Ricky's death. Within another five minutes, I was back on the meditation cushions reciting the memorial service for Ricky. Being able to recite it from memory made it a more powerfully healing experience than reading it could have been.

That vivid experience with intuition should have prepared and warned me to act on another intuition that was equally clear and strong seventeen years later, but it did not. The second intuition was, "Sell the Wellness Center." The Wellness Center was the facility we had built in 1979 to be the home of our holistic medical practice in Albany. Cypress siding, weathered gray, blended harmoniously with stately hundred-year-old pines and massive three hundred-year-old live oaks around the building. From the pine-paneled interior, expanses of glass allowed the eye to enjoy the landscaped grounds. We loved The Wellness Center and loved practicing there. In March 1994, when the intuition came to sell it, I argued, "What do you mean sell The Wellness Center? I love it. I love working here. If I sell The Wellness Center where will I practice?" I chose to ignore the intuition.

April, May and June passed. There was always a low-grade, gnawing awareness that we were where we no longer belonged. I still ignored it. On the second of July a powerful hurricane came ashore on the Florida panhandle and moved north through southwest Georgia and southeast Alabama, dumping about ten inches of rain. It moved into Tennessee, stalled and came back the way it had come, dumping another ten to fifteen inches. At one time, twenty percent of the state of Georgia was under a foot of water. A few days later one percent of the state was under twenty feet of water. That one percent included the Flint River basin and The Wellness Center. Never in recorded history had the land upon which The Wellness Center was built been under water. This time, the water came, and kept coming until it stood five feet deep inside The Wellness Center. In the process, it back-flushed the municipal sewage system into The Wellness Center and the flooded area around it. For two weeks, the Center soaked in sewage solution.

When the water finally went down and we could get back into the building, it was totally devastated. The interior, the patient records, books, computer and most furnishings were destroyed, except for the glass and stainless steel equipment. We had no flood insurance; it had not occurred to anyone that the area would ever flood.

It was a painful lesson, but a valuable one. Not only did it cost us about a quarter of a million dollars, but also substantial time, energy, and emotional suffering. We remembered the proverb, "Experience is a dear teacher, but the only one fools learn by." We learned the lesson well enough not to disregard any clear intuition that has occurred since then.

The flood experience was actually not a total failure to honor intuition. As I walked out of the Wellness Center on the afternoon before it flooded that night, I had a strong intuition to pick up the briefcase containing the notes for this book. I carried it out with me, thus saving many days of work. The notes were the only things I saved from the flood, and they were the most valuable things I could have saved. If I had lost them, I am not sure I would have continued the book project.

The most recent intuitive experience, above the level of the ordinary daily intuitions that I depend on to guide tactical operations, came in March 1997, a few days before my birthday. At that time, we, having taken a hint from nature and moved to the mountains, were developing our new home, Questing Wode, nestled high in a mountain cove. Spring planting season was coming on and we were working diligently to prepare the garden. On the way from the house to the garden each morning, I loaded rocks into the garden cart and stopped by the labyrinth, which a friend had recently outlined. Building the labyrinth was a slow process because the garden cart had a limited carrying capacity. This was of no concern, however, because the focus was on getting the garden ready. Labyrinth construction was a pleasant, brief daily diversion.

Although it was incomplete, I walked through the labyrinth daily, keeping my attention on the question, "What shall I do today to best fulfill my mission?" I always received useful intuitions before I emerged. On this particular morning the intuition was, "Finish the labyrinth ... today!"

I went into my old questioning mode. "What do you mean, finish the labyrinth today? I'm working on the garden, remember? Spring is coming, planting season will soon be here and the garden is not nearly ready."

Something cut the argument short. "Do you need another quarter of a million dollar lesson about what happens when you disregard intuition?"

We could not afford another quarter of a million-dollar lesson. I spent the next hour and a half energetically hauling rock and completing the labyrinth. When the last rock went into place in the last ring of the labyrinth, I felt the energy of the whole area shift into a more coherent, harmonious, powerful configuration. With it, my own energy increased substantially, as did my mental clarity. For the rest of the day I felt more peaceful, had better stamina than I could remember in twenty years, and was more mentally productive. Those benefits have persisted from that day until this. Progress in writing this book accelerated dramatically. I do not know what it would have cost me to disregard that intuition, but I do know it would have taken longer to complete the writing of *Healthspan,* and its quality and usefulness would have been compromised.

What happened that morning? I do not know the whole story, but part of it is that our friend, who designed the labyrinth, told us that one of its functions is to organize energy. He had dowsed the land until he found the most favorable energy configuration for the labyrinth and then marked the outline with gravel. I think the structure immediately started doing what it was supposed to do when its stone structure was completed. I know that I have walked through it at least once almost every day that I have spent at Questing Wode. Every time, I emerge with a better understanding of what I need to do that day to fulfill mission and with more energy to do it.

If you wish to be informed by intuition about what you need to do in order to improve your chances for enjoying the 100-year healthspan and fulfilling your own mission, there are two things that you can do right away. The first is to daily experience the mind-state of quiet alertness. Chopra has called intuition "Nature's intelligence that whispers to us in the silences between our thoughts." In the mind-state of quiet alertness, the silences between thoughts get longer and deeper and it becomes easier to hear the whispers of nature's intelligence. The other thing you can do is to pay attention to your intuitions. A basic law of nature operates here, "Use it or lose it." The corollary is, "Use it and make it stronger."

If you have not had much experience using your intuition, it may not be very reliable at first. It may get confused with what you hope for or fear. It is best to use it on things that are not life-and-death matters until you learn what is intuition and what is something else. As your ability to read your intuition grows stronger and your confidence in it grows, you can rely on it as part of the decision-making process for the most important issues of your life. Intuition and logical reasoning should be in reasonable agreement about what to do, and that is usually the case. However, after collecting the best data you can, thinking it through as clearly as possible, and discussing the issue with people whose judgement you have reason to trust, there may still be a disagreement between reason and intuition. In that case, we encourage you to go with intuition, because you will be right more than ninety-five percent of the time.

Sometimes a patient will tell me of talking to a physician about a strong intuition, backed by past experience, that a different treatment from the one prescribed would be of more benefit. The physician, who evidently thinks M.D. stands for Medical Deity, asks, "How long have you been practicing medicine?"

Perhaps an appropriate response would be, "Not so long, apparently, as you have been practicing arrogance."

ATTENTION AND SYNCHRONICITY (OR CREATING YOUR OWN LUCK)

Mindfulness means putting your attention totally on whatever you are doing now. This is the most difficult way to focus attention—and probably the most powerful. Those who go to the trouble to practice this discipline make discoveries of incalculable value in answering the Three Big Questions. They increase the skill and effectiveness with which they do everything, and often experience fortunate occurrences that they did not expect and were not accustomed to before they began practicing mindfulness. People still mired in the superstition of materialism call these fortunate occurrences luck. Those who have expanded their awareness sufficiently, know that nothing happens by chance because everything is directed by a master intelligence. Those who know this call such occurrences synchronicities.

In my study of Zen Buddhism, I learned about the spiritual discipline of mindfulness, which in Zen is called *tada*. It is highly esteemed as a complementary practice to Zen meditation. For most rapid progress toward enlightenment, Zen recommends that one practice tada all the time one is awake and not meditating. I tried this and found it so useful that I began to prescribe it for some of my patients. A surprising number of them returned to tell me that, soon after beginning the practice of tada, they started having fortunate occurrences that were totally unexpected and unprecedented in their lives. Here are some examples.

Edna was taking her two young sons on a 200-mile automobile trip. They stopped at a roadside park for lunch. After taking the picnic basket out of the car and putting it on a table, Edna noticed steam billowing from beneath the hood of her car. Upon raising the hood, she saw that the radiator hose had broken and was spraying coolant on the hot engine. Since there was nothing she could do about it, she went back to the picnic table and prepared lunch. Just as they were beginning to eat, a man in a pickup truck drove into the roadside park, stopped, and walked over to their table. "It looks like you have a problem, lady," he said.

"It looks like my car has a problem," she replied.

"Well, I think I can fix it for you. Would you like me to do that?"

"Yes, I would."

He got into his truck and drove away. She and the boys ate their lunch. Before they had finished, the man returned with a new radiator hose and some coolant, which he installed. Lunch finished, she repacked the picnic basket and started walking to the car as the man closed the hood. She thanked him and resumed her journey.

George decided it was time to move his family to the country. He put his house on the market and, with a real estate agent, scoured the countryside for suitable property. Months of searching revealed nothing satisfactory. Then, one day he got an excellent offer on his house, provided he would vacate in two weeks. Although he knew there was no suitable property within the distance he could commute, his intuition told him to sell the house. He did so. Within two days, he found the ideal property that months of searching had failed to reveal.

My first encounter with the power of attention was not the end of that story; it never is. The dimension of reality that unfolds to focused attention is limitless and unbounded. It abounds, as I soon discovered, with surprising sequences of synchronicities. From the spring of '75, when I was hurled by terror and distress "through the looking glass" into the awareness of another dimension of reality, until the autumn of that year, I spent some time every day exploring what I called the non-physical universe. I could enter that dimension of consciousness by doing what got me there in the first place: visualizing myself as a tiny speck floating in an infinite universe of love. Once in that dimension of reality, I observed with wonder and delight the freedom, peace, beauty, harmony, and boundlessness that I found there. After discovering that I could move at will between the non-physical universe and the space-time dimension, my functioning in space-time, the world of things and people, improved substantially.

My biggest problem was that I could not find anyone with whom to discuss these adventures. Genevieve was preoccupied with dealing with the havoc I had created in her life, our relationship, and our family during my years of abusing alcohol. It would take a long time for me to rebuild enough credibility with her for her to be ready to listen to my strange adventures in another reality. I tried talking about it with two friends who had told me about their experiences with self-hypnosis to explore, as one of them put it, "the vast space between my ears." I thought they would be more likely than anyone else I knew to understand. When I tried to tell them about these explorations, they responded with uncomfortable silence.

I pursued these adventures alone until October of that year when our family went on its annual leaf season trip. For several years, it had been the family tradition, when the leaves started changing into vivid colors in the southern Appalachians, to take the children out of school, pack the pickup camper and head for the mountains. The children's teachers did not like the week long absences from school, but it was such a fulfilling and delightful experience for all of us that we did it anyway. The children always got their assignments and packed their books, which rested undisturbed in the shelf above the cabover bunk of the camper until our return home a week later.

The autumn of 1975 was an exception. Our older son, Jack III, was working on his assignment to write a comparative study of the world's five great religions. To our astonishment, he continued work during our leaf season adventure until he completed the project. I was so impressed at his unprecedented scholastic diligence that when he finished the project, I asked, "Which of the great religions most closely fits your would view?"

Our fifteen-year-old son replied, "Buddhism."

"Why?" I asked.

"Because Buddhism puts responsibility for one's salvation squarely upon the individual without asking for help from any outside source," Jack III replied.

Hearing his words opened for me a book, *Zen Buddhism*, by D. T. Suzuki. I had bought the book ten years earlier in the Miami airport, because intuition told me there was knowledge there that I needed. I had, however, been unable to read it, so it collected dust on a bookshelf at home for a decade. After hearing Jack III's words I could read it, and did. In that book I learned that what I had discovered about a dimension of reality beyond space-time, others had discovered at least five thousand years ago and had been eloquently and elegantly describing it in depth and detail, writing about it, and living in it, ever since. It was a joy to me to read the experiences and discoveries of many other people.

When I finished the book, I asked our daughter, Marian, who was about to visit a bookstore in another city, to see if she could find another title by D. T. Suzuki. She came back with *The Three Pillars of Zen*, by Philip Kapleau. The bookstore had nothing else by Suzuki. I was disappointed, but since *The Three Pillars* was all I had, I started to read. In Roshi (Zen Teacher) Kapleau's book, I found detailed instructions on how to do the Zen method of focusing attention. I also read descriptions of how others had used this system, zazen as it is known in Zen, to reach this other dimension reliably, sometimes rapidly, and to penetrate it far deeper than I ever had.

One morning in January 1976, I sat down and followed the meditation procedure described by Roshi Kapleau. I meditated for only about five minutes, but when I finished I noticed that my mind was clearer and my energy was better than it had been five minutes earlier. I thought, "Well! If anything can improve my mental clarity and energy in just five minutes, I will do it again."

Sure enough, the next morning the same thing happened. I began to meditate longer and gained still more energy and clarity. The clarity brought with it a peacefulness that, for the first time in my life, set me free from the uneasy feeling that my mind was always fevered, off balance and almost out of control of my will. Doing this meditation was like waking up from a 40-year nightmare. This has been sufficiently valuable to me that I have meditated at least once, and usually twice, a day from that day until this, twenty-four years later.

With regular meditation, my life began to change in the direction of increased peace, productivity, serenity, and compassion. I wrote to Roshi Kapleau, requesting information about how I could learn more about Zen practice. Consequently, I learned about a workshop that the Roshi was giving at the Rochester Zen Center, where he was the abbot. Most of the family went there in November 1976, took the workshop, and learned to do zazen (Zen meditation). I became a student of Roshi Kapleau, and in the next fourteen years benefitted greatly from his teaching.

It took me only a few days in January of 1976 to realize that I wasn't the only person I knew who could benefit from the clarity, energy, and peace I was gaining from doing zazen. Many of my patients who needed those experiences at least as much as I did. I began to teach my psychotherapy patients the Zen method of focusing attention. I had to do this discreetly because I was practicing in southwest Georgia where Zen was generally considered the

Japanese spelling of sin. In as attempt to be politically correct, I called the procedure "mental concentration practice" (MCP).

Remarkably enough, within a few months there was a large room at The Wellness Center dedicated to zazen. The room was often filled with meditators, and no crosses got burned in the front. I took that to be a further manifestation of the power of attention.

ATTENTION AND HEALING EMOTIONAL DISORDERS

As many of my patients began to meditate regularly, I started seeing them make unprecedented progress toward health. A memorable example is that of a woman in her thirties who had such a severe agoraphobia that, in the year before she consulted me, she had left the house three times: once to go to church, once to go to a hospital and once to consult me. She was a prisoner in her own home. Her quality of life was devastated. She had taken the usual drugs for agoraphobic panic; relief had been minimal. I taught her zazen, for which she had a natural aptitude. Within a few weeks, she was more comfortable leaving home to come to The Wellness Center for psychotherapy and meditation.

After meditation one morning she stopped me in the hall and said, "I've had a very strange experience. While I was sitting in the room meditating, suddenly I saw and felt flames all around me. It was terrifying! It took all I could do to keep from jumping up and running out of the room. I remembered what you told me about the possibility that I might have some strange sensory experiences, and if I did, I should keep on meditating because they offered a valuable opportunity for rapid healing. So I sat there and kept on meditating. After a few minutes the flames faded away and with them went my fear of being away form home."

She looked excited. I recognized that she had achieved a powerful healing experience. In the next psychotherapy session a week or two later, she was even more excited. She said that the agoraphobia was completely gone! There was not a trace of it left. She was perfectly free to come and go from her home.

She asked what I thought happened when she was meditating last time. I thought that she had probably recovered a past-life experience that had been causing her agoraphobia. I was not about to say that to a south Georgia farmer's wife, who had probably never heard of past lives, or if she had, believed that such notions were, at best, heathen superstitions. So I said, "I think you recovered a memory and the feelings associated with some terrifying past experience."

She replied, "Yes, that's what happened. I remembered that in my life just prior to this one I was the daughter of my present parents."

I felt a wave of gooseflesh.

She went on, "I was a little girl and had a brother close to my age. One morning he and I were watching mother try to start the fire in the stove by pouring some kerosene on it. I saw flame run up the stream of kerosene from the stove to the spout of the can, which exploded, cutting mother's hands. There was blood and fire everywhere! It was terrifying! My brother and I were terribly burned. Mother took us out and laid us on the front porch. About that time, a neighbor drove by in his pickup truck. Mother screamed for him to stop and help, but he just kept on going.

"After I returned to be their child in this existence, I knew Mother and Daddy didn't like that neighbor, but I never understood why until now. Brother and I died while we were lying there on the porch. My parents were so devastated and grieved so much that I decided to come back again as their daughter to comfort them. Because of this, we have always been very close and loving. When I started meditating, they meditated with me, which helped me a lot. Not long after I was born, they had another son. Then, the family was like it was before the terrible accident."

I never saw that patient again, but a few months later she phoned to tell me that she remained free of agoraphobic symptoms. Her only complaint was that she had sprained her ankle while jogging barefoot on the dirt road in front of her house. I am grateful to that patient for teaching me more than I knew before about the power of attention in activating the self-healing process.

Although few patients achieved healing as dramatic and sudden as this one, the pace of progress for most patients did quicken. Many patients recovered repressed memories and their associated feelings that had been haunting them from outside their awareness. As they brought these memories and feelings into the light of consciousness, health and comfort began to improve. At the same time, I noticed that soon after I began to meditate I was paying the same focused, one-pointed attention to what patients told me in psychotherapy that I paid to counting my breaths, which was the zazen technique I was using at the time. As I began to do this, some remarkable things happened. I found that I could gaze steadily into the eyes of my patients, and could continue to do so with patient after patient, hour after hour throughout the day, At the end of the day, I was far less fatigued and distressed than ever before.

The most impressive thing was that patients I had treated in psychotherapy for two or three years began to tell me things that were deeply painful and shameful to them that they had never mentioned before. Not surprisingly, as they did this, their progress toward health accelerated.

In fact, so many patients told me so much of their pain, suffering, grief and shame that my mind began to feel like a vacuum cleaner, spending each day cleaning one soiled and dusty mind after another. Then, at the end of each day, evening meditation felt like taking the dust bag out of the vacuum and dropping it into a bottomless abyss. I then felt peaceful, relaxed and ready for a refreshing night's sleep—quite a change from the years when I felt so toxic and out of balance from long daily contact with patients that I drank enough alcohol every night to dull my suffering enough to go to sleep.

As I observed all this, my respect and appreciation for the power of attention as a healing modality increased again.

I had gained access to another dimension of reality beyond space-time by focusing attention on visual imagery, but it was meditation that strengthened my power of attention enough to enable me to use the experience of that new (to me) dimension to radically change my life for the better. I also used it to more effectively help my patients. More importantly, the increased power of attention enabled me to more effectively repair the damage I had done to members of my family by my irresponsible behavior during a decade of alcohol abuse.

ATTENTION AND THE BASIS OF HEALTH

When you are sitting on a tack, it takes a lot of Prozac to make that feel good.

—The First Tacks Law of Sidney M. Baker, M.D.

In 1991, I went to Maharishi International University, in Fairfield, Iowa, for two weeks of physician's training in ayurveda. It was the most intensive training and educational experience I had ever had. It felt like four years of medical school in two weeks. At the completion of the training, I went back to the motel, packed my gear into the rental car, and got in to head back to the airport. As I was about to put the key into the ignition, I realized that I had finally learned what I went to medical school thirty-eight years earlier to find out. I had learned in those two weeks the basis, the root cause, of health and disease.

In medical school, I learned much about the mechanisms of disease, but nothing about the *root cause,* and nothing about the cause of health. I learned a lot about how to prescribe the 1950's equivalents of Prozac, but nothing about tack removal—or even that there might be a tack in the first place. In the quest for the answers to these questions, that continued after graduation from medical school, I learned something about what causes health, but the knowledge was fragmentary and there was still nothing about the root cause of disease. To learn that, I had to go to a unique university in a small town in Iowa and study a five-thousand-year-old system of holistic health care.

The basis of health is in balanced awareness

What I had learned was that the basis of health and disease is in consciousness, or awareness. We consider the terms synonymous but prefer *awareness* because *consciousness* has a number of implications beyond what is necessary for health.

To be more specific, the basis of health is in *balanced* awareness and the basis of disease is in *imbalanced* awareness. In order to say what that means in practical terms, I will relate the remarkable piece of knowledge that crystallized the understanding for me. The knowledge is contained in a model discussion that was developed by Maharishi Mahesh Yogi, the founder of the Transcendental Meditation movement and a key figure in the revival of ayurveda, the traditional health care system of India.

The Maharishi begins the discussion by raising the question, "How does your body know how to grow from infancy to adolescence to adulthood? How does your skin know how to heal itself after a wound?" His answer is that it is through nature's own intelligence, which is available in a very practical way to implement whatever healing process is needed. He then points out that disease is caused by imbalances that are the result of certain behaviors, one example of which is overeating. Since all of us at times behave in ways that cause imbalance in our physiologies, restoring the balance becomes vital to regaining and maintaining health.

The discussion goes on to demonstrate in the patient's own experience that there is a state of consciousness in which one is awake and yet does not experience anything except consciousness. This state of consciousness or awareness is best achieved for most people through meditation. In this state of awareness, in which you are awake but experiencing no thoughts or feelings, you are experiencing pure awareness. This pure awareness is the experience of the higher aspect of your Higher Self. A discussion on what Higher Self means is in Chapter 7: Who Am I?

When you are awake, but experiencing no thoughts or feelings, you are awake within yourself. When you are awake within yourself, what you know is your Higher Self. In this state of pure awareness, you are both the knower of yourself and the self who is known. When you are the knower *and* the known, then you must also be the process of knowing. This is a situation in which you are awake and you are the knower, the known, and the process of knowing, so you are one and you are three at the same time.

Unity and diversity

The discussion continues: The oneness, or unity, of the knower, the known, and the process of knowing (or the observer, the observed, and the process of observation) is the reality, and the three are notions of reality developed by the intellect. When awareness is fully alert, the intellect comprehends the unity and the diversity of the three aspects of unity at the same time. In this case, awareness is balanced and this balance, as we shall soon see, is the basis of health. A critical problem arises when the awareness is not fully alert. In this case, the intellect comprehends only the three (knower, process of knowing, and what is known, or the observer, the process of observation, and what is observed). It fails to comprehend the *unity* from which the three aspects came. Since unity is the reality and the three are notions of reality, the intellect has a serious problem: it is suspended on a notion, rather than being aware of reality.

This is a serious problem because the intellect is confronted all the time by an infinitely diverse array of things and situations with which it must somehow deal. Since the Unity from which all of these things emerge has been forgotten, the intellect is unable to see how they are connected and what their true relationship to one another is. Confronted by this appearance of infinite diversity, the intellect feels confused and overwhelmed, like the captain of a ship with a broken compass, caught in a storm at night. The wind drives the ship in one direction; the currents sweep it in another and the captain has not a clue which way to steer because his compass is broken. The best that he can hope for is a frightening, perhaps terrifying, night and the worst he can fear is shipwreck and death.

The mistake of the intellect

This forgetting of the unified basis of life is known in ayurveda as the "mistake of the intellect". Ayurveda maintains that the mistake of the intellect creates an imbalance in awareness that is the root cause of disorder and disease. It is a grievous mistake because it throws awareness out of balance. This is the root cause of disease because, as we saw in the previous chapter, the attention of the observer does something to the object. Balanced awareness has a balancing effect on the body-mind. Imbalanced awareness has an imbalancing effect on the body-mind. When the body-mind system is out of balance, the stage is set for the development of disease. Eventually, in this suboptimal environment in which we all live, disease develops.

The first step in the process of the development of disease in an imbalanced body-mind system is interference with the self-healing mechanism. Balanced awareness activates self-healing; imbalanced awareness weakens it. An active, vigorous self-healing mechanism is essential to the 100-year healthspan.

Overcoming the mistake of the intellect

This raises the crucial question, "How do I overcome the mistake of the intellect and directly experience the unity that underlies all diversity?" You do it through the power of attention. When your power of attention is strong and you focus your attention on your breath, a mantra or whatever enables you to experience quiet alertness, the gaps between your thoughts get wider and wider. What you experience in the gaps between your thoughts is pure awareness, the unity of the observer, the observed and the process of observation. You are already aware of diversity, also known as the diversifying field. That is where all the things and thoughts of your life are. What you experience in quiet alertness, in the gaps between your thoughts, is the unity from which all this diversity came in the first place—and into which it will eventually all return. When your attention is strong enough and focused on the breath, a mantra, or whatever enables you to access pure awareness, the intellect is aware of unity and diversity at the same time. This brings balance to awareness; and through the process of the attention of the observer doing something to the object, it brings balance to the entire physiology. This is the basis of health.

We agree with Myss that there are some exceptions to this rule. She says that some people are sick, not because they are out of balance, but because they have agreed to carry negativity for people who are not strong enough to carry it for themselves. We believe that such instances occur but are relatively rare, and that the vast majority of illness is due to the mistake of the intellect. An illness can be turned into an asset by using it as a stimulus to expand awareness, balance consciousness, and empower the healing process.

Thus, you can see the crucial role that meditation plays in increasing your power of attention enough to enable you to correct the mistake of the intellect. Correcting that mistake balances your awareness, which activates your self-healing mechanism, and maximizes your health, safety, comfort, productivity, and happiness—and the probability that you will attain the 100-year healthspan.

ATTENTION AND STRESS MANAGEMENT

Note: *Genevieve contributed this section.*

One of the first significant pieces of stress management for me came when our older son, Jack III, was about 9 years old. In those days, we did a good bit of camping, either back packing, canoeing, or camping in the pickup camper. Jack had had a welder put together a rack for the pickup that would hold 4 canoes, so we usually had at least three children in addition to our own with us. Sometimes the parents went along also. On this particular canoe trip, we had driven about an hour from home and put the canoes into Lake Blackshear. We then headed north, paddling for about another hour before we stopped and set up camp for the weekend. While I was preparing supper, Jack III stepped on something in the lake that literally laid the bottom of his foot open.

Up until this fateful day, I had always abided by the unspoken rule of how to manage stress in the household in which I grew up: "When in danger—or in doubt—run in circles, scream and shout." Since everything but death and taxes were in the doubtful category, I spent a large amount of my time and energy running in circles, screaming, and shouting.

Jack cleaned J. III's foot as best he could, bandaged it, padded it with a clean white sock, and then put J. III and me into the canoe that had a small outboard motor on it. He told me to get Jack III to the emergency room within two hours; otherwise, the wound would be more likely to get so infected that it might not be possible to put in the sutures that he would need in order to heal properly.

I had never run the motor; I had always paddled. The first thing that I did after we headed back toward the boat landing was to run the canoe into a sand bar. Jack III had to get up on his good foot and help me get the canoe going again. By then I was so tense I could not even think clearly. We finally arrived at the boat dock, got in the VW convertible, and headed toward the hospital. We were running behind time, so I drove that little VW as hard and fast as I could. At some point my guardian angel said to me, "If you continue driving as recklessly as you are driving now, you stand a good chance of killing you, Jack III, and probably some innocent people."

I began to wonder what would be the worst thing that could happen if I did not make the emergency room in two hours. After mulling that over in my mind for a few minutes, I decided that the worst scenario would be that the doctor might have to cut off the foot. That to me was a better option than my killing the two of us — and maybe someone else. With that new knowledge in my head, I started driving at a safe speed. We did not make it to the emergency room in two hours, but the doctor was able to put in the stitches.

That incident set me on a quest to handle the stresses in my life better. Starting on the road to the emergency room, I visualized a graph across my forehead. I called it my worrying scale. It looks like this:

0_____ 50_____100

"0" means that that stress does not amount to a hill of beans. An example might be what I would have for lunch. As long as it is a nourishing lunch, it does not matter a whole lot what I may eat. "50" means that the stress is about halfway between insignificant and a matter of life and death, "100." What I learned about myself while using this scale to "hang all my worries on" was that my body reacted to *all* stresses as if they were a matter of life and death, unless I assigned a number to each situation. An amazing discovery was that most of my "emergencies" do not go higher than 40 on my scale. From that time until this, any time that I feel my guts getting involved in a situation, I immediately try putting the situation on my scale. It works beautifully!

CONCLUSION

We have now considered how the power of attention is the power to gain the freedom and ability to move between two dimensions of reality. Exercising this freedom radically improves functioning in practically every situation, including desperately difficult ones. This empowers you to take control of your life and steer it toward fulfillment, overcome mental and physical health problems, contribute to creating a safer, healthier world, and hone your intuition. We believe that the information in this chapter will increase your understanding of how the power of intuition is the power to attain the 100-year healthspan. Next, Genevieve will tell you how to increase your power of attention.

Help thy brother's boat across, and lo! thine own has reached the shore.

—Hindu Proverb

Chapter 5

STRENGTHENING YOUR POWER of ATTENTION

Having read this far in *Healthspan*, you know that we value the power of attention highly. We believe it is literally the power to claim your birthright and enjoy the 100-year healthspan, starting now. In fact, it is hard to imagine anyone's attaining happiness, high quality of life, and the 100-year healthspan without sufficient power of attention. You probably have some idea by now about some of the reasons we say this. By the time you finish this book, you will know many more. We have observed that most people do not have enough of this power. For all these reasons, we are giving careful attention to the following discussion and instruction on how to strengthen your power of attention.

DISCOVERING MEDITATION

In the late 1970's we purchased *How to Meditate*, by Lawrence LeShan, Ph.D. His observation that, if we had no more control over our bodies than we have over our minds, we would never get across the street, really challenged me. I took his challenge to heart that we try to sit for five minutes without having any thoughts. The harder I tried to keep thoughts out of my mind, the more chatter I heard in my head. I determined to learn to still the mind, to calm it down, to keep it where I wanted it.

First, we learned zazen from Phillip Kapleau. I then attended a seminar by Herbert Benson, M.D. who had devised a meditation for his patients with high blood pressure. He taught us to do what he called, "The Faith Factor." In 1991, we took Transcendental Meditation. All of the above methods are good for helping one calm the chatter in the mind. The important thing is that, whatever system you use, you use it regularly.

GETTING STARTED

There are many different types of meditation, and it is a good thing! No one meditation will fit everyone, any more than my shoes will fit everyone. In this introduction to meditation I will give you the instructions for a type of meditation called by LeShan "the path of the intellect." Zazen, Transcendental Meditation, and Herbert Benson's "The Faith Factor" are examples of the path of the intellect. The other three paths of meditation, according to LeShan, are the path of the body, the path of the emotions and the path of action. Examples of the path of the body are yoga and tai chi. The path of the emotions is the one used by meditators when they are concentrating on loving God or others. The path of action includes such activities as singing hymns, chanting and mindfulness.

Two things many meditations of the path of the intellect have in common are keeping the mind focused on the breath while simultaneously focusing on a word or a phrase, called a mantra. Experienced meditators can meditate just on experiencing breaths. Most beginning meditators, when they try to keep their minds just on breathing, experience what is called the "monkey mind" because the mind seems to jump from thought to thought just as a monkey jumps from tree to tree.

Why keep the mind focused on the breath? Many meditators believe that the breath is where the body and soul meet, or where the physical meets the spiritual. Another way of saying this is that the breath itself carries the Spirit of God within us. It is easier for beginners to keep their minds on the breath *and* a focus word or phrase.

First, find a word of phrase that is meaningful to you, perhaps part of your belief system. (According to an Episcopal Priest, whom we esteem highly, everyone has a religion. He defined religion as man's attempt to make meaning out of an otherwise meaningless existence — or one's attempt to find an ideal way of life.) Robert Schuller, a well known and respected TV evangelist, suggests in his book, *Peace of Mind Through Possibility Thinking*, that Christians use one of the "I Am..." verses in the New Testament as a focus phrase and shorten it to *e om* in order to have a primordial sound. I have found that it is easier for me to keep my attention on a primordial sound than it is to keep it focused on a word such as love or a phrase.

The original primordial sound used as a mantra was *Om* (long "o" as in "ohm"). If you will say this out loud and follow the sound until you are out of breath, you will notice that the sound resonates in your head, thereby helping you to keep focused on it. Ron Roth, a powerful spiritual healer, believes that *Om* is both a manifestation of spiritual power and a symbol of the presence of the Absolute within the material world. Dyer, in his book and tape series, *Manifest Your Destiny*, teaches that *Om* is also the sound of gratitude. Another suggestion of a focus word is "Shalom", usually translated peace; but it also implies wholeness and completeness. It also ends in a primordial sound.

Dr. Benson suggests that we use a phrase such as "Lord Jesus, have mercy on me", or "The Lord is My Shepherd". You will no doubt find a word or phrase that "fits" you. Use that until your intuition tells you that it is time to try another focus word.

Having been raised in a fundamentalist Christian family and educated at a highly respected Christian college, I thought that I had a good understanding of the Scriptures. After reading Ron Roth's new book, *The Healing Path of Prayer*, I realized that what I had been taught was a very narrow, rigid interpretation. The concept of prayer that I had learned and experienced was usually concerned mainly with praising God, asking for forgiveness or asking for help with some problem or asking that He bless/heal other people. In other words, I did all the talking in prayer.

Roth says that the language Jesus spoke was Aramaic. The root word for prayer in that language literally means, "to set a trap". For what are we setting a trap when we pray? Roth says that God is always "broadcasting" love, healing energy, light, love, compassion, and forgiveness. As our minds become still and quiet, we are "tuned" to the frequency through which we can receive the love, healing energy, etc. that God is broadcasting into the world. In other words, we need to stop doing all the talking when we are praying and get the mind still and quiet enough so that we can "catch" the thoughts of God, or let God speak to us. Roth writes: "The most important thing to expect in prayer is contact with God. That is why meditation is so powerful. Unless we are quiet, how can we open our mind to set a trap to catch the thoughts of God? ... The mind in its normal state is never still enough to catch the thoughts of God.... When we enter into prayer, we are recipients of the divine electricity of the Holy Sprit flowing to us upon request."

Read *The Healing Path of Prayer* if you are interested in using prayer as a means of meditation. It is a fascinating book with many suggestions on how to use prayer effectively.

Here are some basic suggestions to help you get started with meditation, whatever path you decide to use:

1. Find a time during the day when you will be undisturbed, such as before the children get up or after they go to bed. Early in the morning (before breakfast unless you have hypoglycemia) and sometime between supper and bedtime are good times. Experiment with what is best for you. It is best to do the meditation at the same time each day if possible.

2. Find a quiet place where you will not hear the TV or stereo. When you get good at this exercise, noise will not bother you;

but make it easy on yourself if you are a beginner. Take the phone off the hook or turn off the ringer. When the body is relaxed in meditation while the mind is alert, noises can be startling. If possible, designate a room or a corner of a room as your meditation retreat. It is helpful to meditate in the same place whenever possible. Our preference for where to meditate is outdoors, when the weather cooperates. We have lived in a quiet, woodsy place for the past 14 years and have enjoyed meditating on the deck or porch. Yes, there are sounds of birds singing and the brook gurgling, but these are natural sounds that are easy to incorporate into the meditation.

3. Get a comfortable, straight chair that is the proper height so that you can keep your spine straight and your feet flat on the floor. Keeping the spine straight helps keep the mind focused.

4. Put a clock where you can see it easily if you are not wearing a wristwatch. Check the time.

5. Close your eyes. Take several deep breaths. While you are breathing deeply, relax your mind; let your thoughts float away as clouds. Next, check the muscles in your body. Tighten and then relax those that are tense. Continue deep breathing until your body is relaxed.

6. When you feel that your body is relaxed, begin breathing normally through your nose. Keep your attention on your breath and your focus word or phrase. When thoughts come into your mind—and they will—gently bring your attention back to your breathing and your focus word. My mother taught me many cliches when I was growing up. One I remember is, "You can't keep birds from flying over your head, but you can keep them from making nests in your hair!" Applying that to meditation, we can not keep thoughts out of our minds, but we can keep from dwelling on them.

Think your focus word(s) on the inhalation or the exhalation. For a two-syllable word such as "e Om" or "shalom", you can say one syllable on inhalation and one on exhalation if you wish. If you say your word or phrase aloud, your voice will probably give out before you have finished meditating. In addition, if you are fortunate enough to have someone meditate with you, it is disturbing to have different people saying different words at different times. (An exception to this would be if everyone is using the same focus word, such as *Om.)*

7. As a beginner meditating alone, start with 10 minutes and build up to 30 minutes twice a day. Decide before you start meditating how much time that you will spend on that meditation. Remember that five minutes spent meditating is better than none at all! When you feel that you have meditated for the time you have set, check your watch or clock. If you had decided to meditate for 20 minutes and you have meditated for only 17 minutes, close your eyes and meditate for 3 more minutes. At the end of the meditation, continue sitting quietly with your eyes closed for another couple of minutes. Then open your eyes and stretch before getting up and going about your business. If you come out of the meditation too quickly, you may not be able to take with you the peace you experienced as you meditated.

As you practice this exercise, you may notice after a few minutes that everything slows. You are not breathing as often; your thoughts do not come as rapidly; most likely, your blood pressure has dropped. It may take several sessions before you become aware of this slowing of the bodily processes.

One word of caution here: Sitting still while meditating does not feel "natural" because we were not brought up to value quiet, still time. In fact, my father told me many times that an idle mind was the devil's workshop. Since I did not want the devil to take up housekeeping in my mind, I made sure it was chattering all the time or I was playing the organ or piano in my head.

Meditating did not feel like a natural thing to do. Now I understand that a meditating mind is by no means idle. In fact, it is working much harder to stay quiet and highly alert at the same time than it is when it is busy chattering.

It takes hard work on our part to keep the body still and the mind meditating when we were not brought up to value that kind of activity. Hang in there! After several weeks, you will begin to feel more peace in the stillness than you ever felt in the harried state in which most of us live.

When Benson was doing the research that led to his teaching "The Faith Factor Meditation" to his patients with high blood pressure, he found that the meditators did indeed lower their blood pressure while meditating. However, he also found that the body exhibited the exact opposite of what it experiences when it is in the flight/flight mode. In order to live creative, healthy lives, we need to dissipate stress as rapidly as possible so that it does not accumulate in the body. Exercising and meditating regularly are two efficient ways to de-stress the body/mind. Of course, the two methods for defusing stress that are the most enjoyable are having sex and laughing. Unfortunately, those two methods are not always appropriate or available to us. Physical exercise and meditation, however, are available to us a good bit of the time, if we but choose to use them.

I had an especially hard struggle getting myself to meditate. I was brought up at a time when it was the woman's place to take care of all the needs of the family except for making the living; that was the responsibility of the male. Since the housework, laundry, cooking, etc. were never caught up, I felt guilty taking time to be still and quiet and spend time on myself. I felt guilty for not being up and busy taking care of three active children and a home in addition to working outside the home. In my generation, the unspoken rule was that females take care of other people; they do not take care of their own needs.

When you are using this technology of quiet alertness for twenty to thirty minutes every day, some remarkably beneficial and pleasant things will begin to happen in your life. Increased energy, mental clarity, and peacefulness are the ones that are likely to appear first. When you begin to *commit* twenty to thirty minutes twice a day to the process, the benefits more than double and you begin to experience the extraordinary healing power of quiet alertness, because you will have strongly activated your self healing mechanism.

Although many beneficial things will happen, there may also be difficulties and unpleasant experiences associated with the meditation or, as Jack prefers to call it, the quiet alertness technology. For one thing, your ego will rage against it because your ego knows that you are directly experiencing that which is incomparably greater than ego. As we will explain in subsequent chapters, ego will do everything possible to keep you from going forward with this increase in your power of attention. Jack remembers that in the first year he was practicing meditation, he had to struggle with his ego before practically every time he sat down to meditate —and that was twice a day. His ego would go into frenzy against what he was about to do, saying, "You fool! How could you even consider doing anything so stupid as meditation when there are so many important, pleasant, interesting, fun and useful things you could be doing?" That communication from ego was always accompanied by a feeling of revulsion against meditation. In spite of all that, he went ahead and did it anyway because he had directly experienced the energy, mental clarity, and peacefulness that always flowed into his life because of meditation. Ego, for all its promises, had never, ever delivered anything even approaching such value.

Eventually, after about seven years, ego gave up and began to serve the quiet alertness process. In the last decade, his emotional response to the prospect of meditation has been one of longing and eagerness because, as Lawrence LeShan wrote, "It's like coming home." It's not only *like* coming home: it *is* coming home. The Field of Pure Consciousness is our true home, as we will discuss in Chapter 7, "Who Am I?". It is where we came from in the first place and where we will eventually return after we have done everything we need to do, played out all the roles we want to play out, and exhausted all our karma during however many cycles of existence are necessary to accomplish all that. In the meantime, once you have sufficient power of attention, you can visit your true home anytime you wish and return from the visit invigorated and refreshed, with better balance and mental clarity to deal with whatever you need to deal with in ordinary waking consciousness.

Another experience that may be a problem as you build your power of attention is the return to consciousness of repressed memories and feelings. These can take the form of some strange, uncomfortable, and even frightening sensory experiences. The case of a woman who recovered from agoraphobia, about whom you have already read, is an example of this.

For an explanation of how repressed memories still dictate many of our actions and moods, read Dr. Thomas Harris's best seller, *I'm OK; You're OK*. In this book, he details the studies that established that at least at birth, and probably before birth, a child starts a two-level recording of all her experiences. She records in detail what happened (the memory of the event) and what her feelings of the event were.

If it was a painful experience, she no doubt learned to repress the memory of the event. Repressing the feeling that went along with the event, however, is impossible. The feeling continues to "play" at times, influencing our relationships, our decisions and certainly our moods. Reconnecting the memory of the event with the feeling experienced in the event sets us free as adults to rethink the situation, process it in the light of our mature knowledge, and free ourselves of unwanted intrusions of inappropriate feelings.

During the first year that Jack was meditating, some very angry feelings came back into his awareness. During that time, he had to be careful not to express the anger to people around him. He knew that if he simply let it come into awareness and continued his meditation practice it would dissipate—and it did. At the end of that time, he was wonderfully free of anger and resentment. He was able to deal skillfully and calmly with situations to which he would have previously reacted by going into a rage and doing destructive things.

AVOIDING THE TAR BABY TRAP

In *The Complete Tales of Uncle Remus*, Joel Chandler Harris wrote a delightful cautionary tale about how Br'er Rabbit's penchant for judging and coercion put him in the clutches of Br'er Fox, who dearly wanted to have Br'er Rabbit over for dinner. A tar baby was the RSVP invitation. When the tar baby failed to respond to a friendly "Good morning!", Br'er Rabbit elected to teach him manners by punching him. Soon, Br'er Rabbit's hands were stuck fast. Realizing that he was in a dangerous situation, he tried to make the tar baby release him by first kicking and then butting. Eventually he was stuck so tightly that he had no choice but to accept Br'er Fox's invitation to dinner. How Br'er Rabbit extricated himself from that predicament is another story—a charming one that you would probably enjoy reading for yourself.

Meditators, particularly *beginning* meditators, get stuck in a similar trap when they try to keep thoughts out of their minds while meditating. There is a pervasive belief that for meditation to be effective, the mind must be kept blank, free of thought. Fortunately, that is not true, but we find that more people have trouble with this trap than with most other aspects of meditation. Patients often say, "I'm not doing well with meditation. No matter how hard I try to keep thoughts out of my mind, they just keep coming. I'm discouraged."

We then remind them that the object of meditation is to quiet and focus the mind and strengthen the power of attention, *not* to keep thoughts out of the mind. It is very rare that anyone gains sufficient power of concentration to do that for more than a few moments. Many people want to do so, though. The issue has been around for a long time. A Zen poem addresses it:

Though still waters range to the vast blue autumn sky
How can they compare to the hazy moon on a spring night?
Most people desire pure clarity
But sweep as you will, you cannot empty the mind.

The benefits come from doing the meditation procedure correctly and regularly, not from keeping thoughts out of the mind. Trying to keep thoughts out of the mind only invites more to come in. It is as counterproductive as Br'er Rabbit's trying to make the tar baby release him by striking it. Instead, when you realize that you are thinking instead of focusing your attention on your mantra or breath, just say silently and gently to yourself, "Oh, well," and go back to focusing on your meditation.

MEDITATION GROUPS

When you are learning meditation and incorporating it into your lifestyle, it is helpful to sit with a meditation group whenever you can. Daily would be ideal, but even once a week is a great help. A group of people using this technology together at the same time creates an energy field that makes it easier for everyone to strengthen attention more quickly and deeply. If you live in a city, there are probably many meditation groups. If you do not know where any of them are, you might check with a Unity Church or a TM or Zen Center. People who go to Unity are likely to appreciate the importance of meditation, and there may be one or more groups sitting at the church.

Whenever and wherever you join a meditation group, be wary of the guru trap. There are many people who are offering to lead others on their spiritual journeys. Some of these gurus can be helpful, but others, who may be charismatic, can lead one into disasters such as the Jonestown massacre, the Branch Davidian catastrophe, and the Heaven's Gate mass suicide. When Deepak Chopra was on "Larry King Live", Larry asked him how it felt to be the guru for so many people. Dr. Chopra replied that he felt each person ought to be his/her own guru. He then asked Larry to spell guru, which Larry did. Chopra said, "See? Gee! You Are You."

When your power of attention is strong enough, you will be able to access the Field of Pure Consciousness. When you can access Pure Consciousness, you will find the right answers to every problem and question in your life. Once you can do this, you do not need any guru to tell you what to do. You know what to do, because "Gee! You Are You!"—and you know who this you is, why you are here and what is the true nature of your relationships to the other people in your life. Quite a lot of benefit from something so simple as meditation!

DEVELOPING AN ATTITUDE OF GRATITUDE

Let us mention one of the most important types of meditation on the path of the intellect—gratitude. One of the best ways to stay healthy mentally, physically, and spiritually is to develop an attitude of gratitude. Many of us were brought up to say a prayer of gratitude before we begin eating a meal. That is great, but three times a day is hardly enough to keep our minds focused on what we *have*, not on what we *lack*. As we slowly awaken to each new day (hopefully without hearing an alarm clock!), it is helpful to verbalize our gratitude at coming safely through another night and having a whole new day full of opportunities and challenges.

There was a popular song when we were teenagers about counting our blessings instead of sheep when we had problems sleeping. Going to sleep with gratitude in our hearts and on our minds is a wonderful transition from wakefulness to sleep.

I started having major problems falling asleep after my favorite neighbor died when I was 5 years old. When I looked out my bedroom window on that warm summer night after Mrs. Brown died, I could see her body in the casket in front of the her living room window. This was a highly disturbing scene to my five-year-old eyes. Dad tried to placate me by telling me that dying was like going to sleep. Since I did not want to get put into a box and put in the ground, I unconsciously decided that it was not smart to go to sleep. As I grew up, I found that meticulously verbalizing my blessings helped me to calm down and get ready for sleep. I started by being grateful for a clean bed, warm covers, a clean floor to put my feet on, and so forth. As the family began camping, I learned to be grateful for even more things — hot water, a bathtub, inside plumbing, a roof over our heads, etc. There is no end of things for which to be grateful. Often now, when I have difficulty dropping off to sleep or wake up during the night and have problems going back to sleep, I just say over and over again, "Thank You!"

It helps to set aside some time each day just to concentrate on our blessings. When we are teaching seminars, we suggest that our students write down at least five things each day for which they are grateful. Most people find that they can literally fill pages! The important point here is to make gratitude an important part of every day. Having certain times to concentrate on blessings is helpful. Driving to work can be used as a time of gratitude. Walking for exercise is a great time to be grateful for legs that work well, time to exercise, etc. Find several times each day to count your blessings. Remember that what you keep your attention on expands in your life!

ADVANCED TECHNIQUES

As your power of attention strengthens through practice of the techniques described here, you will come to a plateau. You will then find yourself wanting to go past that point; you will need an advanced technique. When that time comes, we encourage you to read about zazen in *The Three Pillars of Zen,* by Roshi Philip Kapleau. If you are using prayer as a meditation, Ron Roth has useful information on how to improve your meditation. He also teaches seminars. For further information about his seminars, call Celebrating Life Institutes listed in Resources.

While learning any technique for strengthening the power of attention, it is a great help to have a skilled teacher. This is particularly true with zazen. Many cities have Zen Centers that offer such instruction. If you do not have access to a good instructor, you can still make effective use of the clear, precise, detailed instructions in *The Three Pillars of Zen*. As you may recall from the previous chapter, this was Jack's entry point into strengthening the power of attention. In fact, he did zazen for fourteen years. He then learned Transcendental Meditation because it was the technique associated with ayurveda, which he was studying. Transcendental Meditation served him well for seven years. Then, when he came to the most difficult part of writing this book, he realized that he was going to have to strengthen the power of attention further in order to complete the book. He resumed doing zazen, which gave him greater power of attention because the technique calls for sitting with the spine unsupported and erect and the eyes open. Keeping the eyes open increases alertness. It also increases distractions, so one sits in front of a blank, neutral colored wall or screen. Sitting with the spine erect immediately gives better control over the mind, making it possible to attain more quietness. Thus the magical combination of quietness and alertness was enhanced; the power of concentration increased and the writing process went forward again.

In his valuable and fascinating audiocassette album, *Magical Mind, Magical Body*, Chopra describes a test to determine whether the technique you are using is right for you. He asks four questions. "Did your mind find the quietness it was seeking? Was the meditation psychologically comfortable to you? Did the meditation change you in the direction in which you wish to change? Is there more truth in your life because you meditated?" If you can answer those four questions affirmatively, the technique you are using is right for you, whatever it is. We suggest that you do not try to answer these questions until you have been meditating regularly for at least one month.

TECHNOLOGY FOR ACCELERATING THE PROCESS

Sufficient power of attention is essential in two ways for the attainment of the 100-year healthspan. We have already considered how the power of attention can be used to balance awareness, which is the basis of health because it activates the self-healing mechanism of the body-mind.

The other thing that makes sufficiently powerful attention essential is that it permits the expansion of awareness to include more knowledge. As Albert Einstein observed, "The significant problems we face cannot be solved at the same level of thinking we were at when we created them." The power of attention is the power to expand awareness to a higher level than the one that existed when the problem was created. Once you do that, you have opened the possibility of solving the problem that would otherwise be insoluble.

If you recall the chapter on Dream Destroyers, you are aware that humankind faces some daunting problems, a combination of which could conceivably end the tenure of the human race on earth, or at least destroy civilization as we know it. If humankind did not actually perish, it could return to a level of existence that has been described as nasty, brutish and short—hardly the 100-year healthspan that is nature's birthright to us. There is ample evidence that, if you persistently and consistently use the technologies already described in this chapter, you will reliably strengthen your attention. You can then use this greater strength to achieve higher levels of awareness that empower you to solve your previously unsolvable problems.

Historical records and everyday experience make it clear that where the deepest, most difficult problems are concerned, this process usually takes years. At this crucial point in human history, we probably do not have years. For humankind to solve the potentially lethal problems it confronts, masses of people must achieve higher levels of awareness far more quickly than history indicates is possible. Here technology can be of great assistance and can actually make the difference between humankind's doing the pull-up to a higher level of consciousness and evolution or drifting down to a much lover one.

The technology is called neurofeedback. It grew out of biofeedback, but is a quantum leap beyond it. Neurofeedback provides information about brain activity rather than body activity such as skin temperature, muscle tension, and heart rate. One form of neurofeedback enables one to read his brain wave activity on a monitor and/or hear auditory signals that indicate different types of brain activity. With this feedback, one learns what to do with one's mind in order to rapidly strengthen the power of attention and expand awareness.

Another form of neurofeedback uses brain activity to drive lights to flash at frequencies one hertz faster or slower than the dominant brainwave frequency. This disentrains or extinguishes old maladaptive neural patterns and circuits. It simultaneously activates latent neural circuits that have never been used before. These newly activated circuits can then be programmed to do whatever one wishes them to do. By using these technologies, it is possible for most people to achieve power of attention and balanced awareness in weeks or months that previously took years or decades. This opens the possibility for enough people to achieve enough expansion of awareness to create a new social consciousness that will permit the solution of dream destroying problems that are insoluble at our present level of awareness: violence, drug abuse, racial hatred, pollution, poverty and the health care crisis.

When we moved to Rabun County, we were fortunate to meet the neurofeedback practitioner who discovered and published the first paper on the ability of neurofeedback to expand awareness. His pioneering work at Woodridge Hospital has opened the door to recovery from substance abuse and relief of intractable, disabling pain for many people. Marty Wuttke invited Jack to experience the neurofeedback technology. What he experienced was that in a twenty-minute session he could gain the clarity and expanded awareness that previously required a week in a Zen meditation retreat.

Given the necessity of sufficient power of attention and balanced, expanded awareness to achieve a high quality of life and the 100-year healthspan, we encourage everyone to consider using the neurofeedback technology.

In Resources, you will find a telephone number for the national referral services to neurofeedback practitioners. If you consult one, it is important that you tell him or her that your objective is to strengthen your power of attention and expand your awareness as rapidly as possible. Neurofeedback is used for many purposes. If your provider knows exactly what your expectations are, he/she can devise the protocol that will be most time efficient and cost effective. Since practitioners vary widely in skill, knowledge, and experience, we encourage anyone for whom it is feasible to have a consultation with Mr. Wuttke, who pioneered the whole process and is more knowledgeable about it than anyone else we know. In a recent conversation, he told Jack that he is now working on protocols to be used in a brain mapping system that is likely to accelerate the process another quantum leap above where it is now. If this technology fulfills its potential, it may enable most people to accomplish in weeks what it previously took decades to do. Mr. Wuttke's telephone number is also listed in Resources. He is no longer working at Woodridge Hospital; he is now the director of the Institute for Family Wellness in Atlanta.

CONCLUSION

The benefits of learning to keep the mind calm and focused are many. I would like to share with you two success stories:

"The New Age Journal" reported several years ago the account of a woman whose lover, a previous drug user, had already died from AIDS. She also had the virus and knew that her time was limited. She was house sitting at the time. She spent many hours each day meditating to get herself ready to make the transition into the next existence. After doing this for several months and experiencing a radical expansion of awareness, she realized that she felt much better. She asked her physician to re-check her for AIDS. The virus was totally gone! The physician said that she had obviously been misdiagnosed. (This is a fre-quent response from physicians whose patients disobey their prognoses.) Please note that she was not trying to heal herself!

The second account was reported in one of Bernie Siegel's books, probably *Love, Medicine, and Miracles*. A RN had an in-curable, progressive disease. Her body had deteriorated so much that she was wheelchair bound. She decided that she would not die until she had learned to love her body. Each day she took off her clothes, sat in front of a mirror, and concen-trated on loving a part of her body. One day she concentrated on loving her hand; another day it was a foot, etc. Over a period of time her functioning improved so that she was no longer con-fined to a wheelchair. She was able to resume a normal life. Please note that this person, also, was not trying to heal herself. Her concentration was on learning to love herself.

Some of the benefits of learning to keep the mind focused include:

1. A feeling of oneness with the universe and other people, thereby dispelling fear

2. Improvement in personal relationships

3. Lower blood pressure

4. Weight loss for the overweight (losing one's addiction to food)

5. Improved performance (some teams meditate before go-ing on the field to play football, etc. People have also im-proved their golf games) at work, play or home.

6. Ability to set priorities, thereby eliminating many unnec-essary activities in our lives

7. Better handling of stress, especially during crises

8. Management of physical pain

9. Improved outlook on life, ability to see positive results while in the midst of emotional, physical, spiritual or financial stress.

10. Healing painful memories of past experiences

11. Learning to keep the mind focused on the here and now.

There are many other benefits; these will vary from individual to individual based on how disciplined one is in regularly and wholeheartedly doing some meditative practice.

This strengthening of the power of attention is probably the most important thing you will ever do to achieve the 100-year healthspan and happiness along the way. We tell our patients, "Ruthlessly protect your meditation time." It is the most loving thing you can do for yourself and everybody else.

Never pay attention to what critics say. Remember, a statue has never been set up in honor of a critic.

—Jean Sibelius

Chapter 6

WHO AM I? WHY DON'T I KNOW?

Who am I? is the only question worth asking and the only one never answered.

— Deepak Chopra, MD, in *The Way of the Wizard.*

INTRODUCTION

In order to have your best chance to experience the 100-year healthspan and the highest quality of life every day from now until then, you either have to have the answers to The Big Questions or you have to be in the process of answering them. The Big Questions are: Who am I? Why am I here? What is the true nature of my relationship to these other people in my life? The answers to the second and third questions come easier if you have the answer to the first one. The answer to each of these questions is not just any answer; it is *your* answer. Nobody else can answer the question for you. Other people can tell you how to find your answer, but nobody can find it and give it to you.

If you are in New York and you want to be in San Francisco, no one else can go there and give you the experience of being there. We can tell you how to get to San Francisco, but you still have to act on that knowledge in order to have the experience of being in that beautiful city. We can, and will, tell you how to discover your real, true self, but you have to act on that knowledge if you are to have an experience incomparably more wonderful, thrilling and delicious than anyone could ever have by going to San Francisco—or anyplace else.

In this chapter, we will first explain why so few people know who they really are, then why it is important to know. In Chapters 7 and 8, we will discuss how to find out.

WHY DON'T I KNOW?

Discovery of one's true self is so difficult and so little appreciated in our culture dominated by the superstition of materialism that most people abandon the quest during adolescence. This is a crucial and tragic mistake. It is like coming to a fork in a path and taking the one that leads to a life of quiet desperation, mediocrity, and regret. The other fork, "the road less traveled by," leads to high adventure, fulfillment, happiness, and the 100-year healthspan. We invite you to return to this crucial fork and take the path that leads to your own personal, valid, viable answer to the first big question. The decision to follow this path is not one that most people take lightly. It looks like a path that will demand strenuous exertion—and it will. It is hard to see at the point at which you have to make the decision that the rewards will be greater than the effort. The only reason that anyone chooses the hard path is probably a deep knowing that it is the only one that leads to happiness and fulfillment.

Why should discovery of one's true self require effort and self-discipline? We identify five reasons.

- The condition of childhood
- The dirty-water brainwash
- The superstition of materialism
- The mistake of the intellect
- The mistake of the ego

The condition of childhood

Thomas Harris, M.D., in his landmark book, *I'm OK: You're OK*, acquaints us with what he calls the situation of childhood.

Most parents begin the "civilizing" process on their children just as soon as the child is old enough to learn that many of her actions will not be acceptable when she goes to grandmother's house or when she goes to play school. Things that come naturally to the child—such as wetting one's pants when the bladder is full, screaming when unhappy, eating with fingers instead of with a spoon or a fork—are often "corrected" by the parent or care giver, or even punished. Over the period of the first few years, the messages that the child hears most often are "No!" or "Don't touch that" or something similar.

By the time the child is 5 years old, he has within his head a whole list of acceptable and unacceptable behaviors. Children are born wanting to please the big people in their lives. They do not like to experience pain from discipline, whether it is physical or emotional. Harris makes a good point that we decide very early in life, before we have developed the brain and experience to make good decisions, that we are not OK but that the big people are OK. The next big question is, "What must I do in order to keep the big people around to take care of me?" The answer to that question is always, "Adapt! Adapt! Adapt! " Those of us who were brought up by strict parents pretty much lost our identity, our true self, before we started to school. Our lives from that point onward are concerned with pleasing other people — first our parents, then our teachers, peers, employers, spouses, etc.

How, then, does one raise children who are "acceptable" to society if the care givers do not do the "civilizing" process? We decided when our children were small that we would not teach them manners; instead, we would always treat them with respect and would use good manners around them. This drove their grandparents wild. The Woodards, the only grandparents who lived in easy driving distance, tried to keep the two oldest children for several days at a time so that they could teach them what we were failing to teach. By the time our daughter was five years old, she had learned to dial long distance and ask us to go pick her up. She had had all the "civilizing" she could stand! Did our experiment work? A big, resounding "YES". We never asked them to answer adults as sir and ma'am, but they discovered at school that the teachers liked being addressed that way, so they picked it up naturally. Our daughter was about 9 years old before she asked how to cut her meat with a knife and fork. Until that time, she just did it as best she could.

The point we would like to make here is that children learn much better from example than they do from demands that they act a certain way. By the time our children were school age, they had good manners — naturally. We believe that the key to good manners is respect. When Gen asked me what would be the best time to start toilet training our first child, I replied, "When she can say, 'Mother, I need to urinate'". It worked. She never had to go to play school in diapers!

Unfortunately, most children were frequently "corrected" when they did not conform to the norm that our civilization dictated, so the child grew up thinking that all his natural tendencies are bad; therefore, he is bad, not OK. Since the part of him that is "natural" is no good, it is best that he discount that part of himself and adapt to the demands of civilization. Because of this, many children grow up with low self esteem and thus spend their time and energies trying to do those things that will get them praise, not discomfort or punishment. Others, if pushed too far, rebel and become antisocial. Neither of these responses is conducive to the individual's knowing who he or she is.

A natural extension of the condition of childhood is the condition of adolescence. It presents its own set of challenges for adolescents and for their parents. The challenges are different, but no less rigorous. For parents, they may seem more difficult. The passage through adolescence has been called getting over fool's hill. Wayne Dyer wryly refers to it as the age of demonic possession. The perils of the process for adolescents themselves are indicated by the rising rate of violence, including murder and suicide.

One of the most important challenges as we start through puberty is to answer the question, "Who am I, separate and apart from my parents?" If we live with both biological parents and know relatives on both sides of the family well, we have a good start. If our parents encourage our learning to think for ourselves (within reason, of course!), we get a little closer to answering our question. If, on the other hand, every time the young person voices an opinion that is contrary to what the parents think, they nearly go into orbit, the developing adolescent may be discouraged from ever finding out how he is a separate, unique human being. What happens to many adolescents, who are exploring this territory, is that they rebel and do the opposite of what the parents do. There is no freedom in rebellion. They are still "stuck" in the family system, but doing the opposite. If parents have the skills and patience to help steer the adolescent through these stormy seas, the tension level between parents and teenagers will be very low. More about how to do that in the forthcoming book on relationships. Fortunate indeed is the adolescent who gets support from parents in his quest for his answer to the first big question while he is still at home!

Brainwashed with dirty water

All your life you have been hearing other people tell you who you are. All your life they have been giving you misinformation and disinformation about who you are. At best, those who have been telling you do not know. At worst, what they have been telling you is what they believe will give them power over you, so that they can manipulate you to do what they want done. In this sort of disinformation the essential message is, "You are weak, helpless, stupid, bad, ugly, foolish, and disgusting. You had better do what I tell you, or I will abandon you and you will suffer and die." The message usually is not that clear and direct, but it sounds like something that you heard in the condition of childhood. In that condition, the threat had considerable power. On an unconscious level it still does. People who know how to push that button of yours can have great influence upon you. Until you know your true self and know that you know, you are susceptible to brainwashing with dirty water. All of us have had our minds shaped by approximately 25,000 hours of pure conditioning, all of which comes from people who do not know who we are. Most of the conditioning comes from people who do not care who we are, but do care about manipulating us into doing what they want done. Considering this can begin to provide an idea of the magnitude of this problem.

A more subtle and perhaps even more dangerous aspect of not knowing your true self is that there are people who tell you that you are wonderful, beautiful, smart, and powerful. If you like hearing this, all you have to do in order for them to keep on telling you is do what they want you to do. If you do not know who you really are and are desperate to hear somebody say something nice about you, this kind of subtle manipulation may be even more effective, and therefore more troublesome, than the kind that is powered by derogatory statements. Most people get both kinds. The carrot and the stick move the donkey more effectively than either one alone.

The superstition of materialism

Our culture is still in the grip of the superstition of materialism. We are all controlled by it to one degree or another. That superstition says, "If you can't see it, touch it, smell it, taste it or hear it, it isn't real." The most important part of who you are, your spirit, cannot be perceived by any of the senses. The superstition of materialism, therefore, asserts that your spirit does not exist. This gives you a choice. You can believe the superstition, as most people do, and forget about discovering who you are, or you can choose to free yourself from the superstition by believing your heart and your intuition, which know beyond doubt that there is more to you than your body. Read about how to do that in the next chapter.

It is not easy to break free of a dominant cultural superstition. People who believe and live the superstition feel threatened by those who do not. When people feel threatened, they are likely to either withdraw or attack. Neither response is comfortable, particularly if the other person is important to you or attacks with intensity. Thus, the superstition is a potent force blocking the way to self-discovery. Fortunately, there are potent counterforces available, but they are not for the faint-hearted.

The mistake of the intellect

In Chapter 4, there is a discussion of "the mistake of the intellect," which is ignorance of the unified basis of life. You probably recall that ayurveda considers it the basis of disease. It is also another potent obstacle to knowing your real self. The fully alert intellect is aware of both the things of the material world and the unity from which they all came. Since the highest aspect of your true self is this unity, you have to overcome the mistake before you can know who you are. Instructions on how to do that are in Chapter 4.

The mistake of the ego

The fly sitting on the hub of the chariot wheel looked back and exclaimed, "Lo, what a dust I raise!"

—Ancient proverb

Ego is a problem that must be understood and solved if you are to discover who you are. Ego is like fire: a useful servant but a fearful master. We use the term *ego* in the popular sense, as when one says, "She is egotistical," or "He has a big ego." Chopra defines ego as all our ideas about who we are. He says, "It is the collectedness of all the things we identify with. People collect the totality of their labels, their ideas and concepts in the intellect. They say, *"That's me!"* That's the ego—just a figment of the imagination."

A figment of the imagination indeed, but what a powerful figment! Ego always has incurable "more" disease. No matter how much you have, ego wants *more*: more power, more admiration, more pleasure, more money, and more security, more of everything. Ego is always demanding more because it is based on illusion rather than reality. Ego comes into existence out of the necessity for human consciousness to organize and understand experience.

Without an organizing function in consciousness, there would be consciousness only of chaos. A planned and organized life would be impossible. Meher Baba, a prominent Indian spiritual teacher, observed that the ego functions like the ballast of a ship. The ballast gives the ship stability, protecting it against capsizing from the action of wind and waves. The ego is necessary to the functioning of consciousness, but it is a necessary evil. The evil is the fundamental mistake that the ego makes as it comes into existence in the early life of each person. The mistake is that the ego begins with the false idea that it is the physical body. This makes it inevitable that the ego feels separate from the rest of life. It also makes it inevitable that the ego deny the importance, and sometimes even the existence, of the spirit. This is a tragic mistake because spirit *is* real, *is not* the physical body, and is the only basis for fulfilling the longing for peace, security, joy, love, and completeness.

Since ego has established itself on an illusion (that it is the body and separate from everything and everyone else), it can only build one illusion atop another. Thus, it must feel increasingly insecure, unstable, and incomplete. It tries to relieve its insecurity and emptiness by getting more and more external objects to promote the illusion that it is real. "See," it says, " I have all these things, all this admiration and praise from other people, all this power, all this money. That proves that I'm real."

However, it does not; it never can, because what is real is something else. That real something else, spirit, is forever beyond the reach of the ego, because the ego was established on and can never move beyond the false belief that it is the physical body and separate from everything else in creation. The ego's falseness condemns it to perpetual frustration and disappointment. Perpetual frustration and disappointment engender craving, hatred, anger, fear, and jealousy. These attitudes cause massive problems in relationships and complications in life. The resulting stress and anxiety, to say nothing of violence, are deadly hazards to quality of life and the 100-year healthspan. In addition, who would want to live 100 years with these attitudes and experiences, even if it were possible to stay physically healthy for that long?

Fortunately, there is an alternative to living an ego-ridden life. You can directly experience what is the real you and directly know the security, carefreeness, lightheartedness and laughter that comes with that knowing, and from being truly secure at last. Although you can meet, recognize, know, and be your true self, ego will do everything it can to keep you from it. Ego will fight it tooth and nail because it knows that once its falseness is unmasked, it will lose its power. Once you see behind the curtain, as Dorothy did when she confronted the terrible Wizard of Oz, ego will have to become the servant of your spirit rather than the master of your body-mind. To ego, this is worse than death, so it will give you a full demonstration of its power and cunning. It will delay, but cannot prevent, your finally meeting your Whole Self and knowing the joy of that ultimate wholeness and authentic power.

In practical terms, ego is likely to try to get you to believe that there is no validity to any of this knowledge that you are now gaining. It will try to make you believe that it cannot possibly work, and that you would be stupid even to try it to see. It will insidiously insist that the only safe thing is to trust ego and believe it is the highest aspect of you. Ego will try to frighten you into believing that only it can protect you from destruction. It will warn that in order to survive you must keep up the desperate struggle to get more money, power, admiration, security, and pleasure. Ego is powerful and convincing, but you can override it. You can do so because you know at the deepest level of your awareness that what you are learning is true and that you can discover and be your true self.

When you begin this process, you will experience increasing energy, mental clarity, inner peace, and personal power. This will feel wonderful and will bring you comfort, strength, and security that following ego's orders never did and never can. It will also spur ego to even more desperate attempts to throw you off this track. You may, for example, experience the return of old feelings of guilt, fear, and self-doubt. Ego can do this. Whenever you have a setback in your progress, as all of us do from time to time, ego will jump in with great ferocity and say, "See, you are a total failure. I told you from the beginning this couldn't work. Now go back to doing what I tell you, because I am the only one you can trust and the only one who can protect you against terrible suffering and destruction." Like the wizard of Oz, ego can produce frightening illusions that look real until you have the courage to yank the curtain aside and see the pathetically feeble creature hidden behind it. The ultimate solution to solving the problem of ego is to meet, greet, know, and be your Whole Self.

In the meantime, be warned that ego will fight ferociously to stay in control of your life. It will play many tricks to deceive you into believing that there is no higher authority or intelligence. Of all the obstacles to discovering who you are, ego is usually the most formidable. In Chapter 13, we will tell you how to find the knowledge, power, and grace to master this worthy adversary, make it your servant, and eventually to dispense with it entirely.

WHAT DOES IT MATTER WHETHER OR NOT I KNOW WHO I AM?

Since it is probably going to require some significant effort for you to find your own valid, satisfying, reliable, useful answers to this first big question, we have a responsibility to tell you what will make it worth your time and effort. Actually, we have already presented some of this in Chapters Three and Four, but this particular knowledge is so crucial that a brief review is worthwhile.

Ignorance causes a cascading concatenation of calamities

The most enlightened and wise people who have ever lived have reached a consensus that ignorance is the worst curse of humankind. Of all forms of ignorance, unawareness of one's true nature is the most dangerous. It slams the door on the 100-year healthspan and lasting happiness while opening the gate to untold suffering. Here are some of the mechanics by which it happens.

Anxiety and depression are mortal enemies of the 100-year healthspan. Excess free radicals and a suppressed immune system are also mortal enemies of the 100-year healthspan. If you have a lot of anxiety, you have an excessive number of free radicals. If you have an emotional depression, you have immune system depression. Free radicals rip and tear cell membranes, damage tissue, and are the final common pathway of disease and premature aging. A depressed immune system is unable to adequately defend you against infectious disease and cancer. There are also some immune system disturbances, called autoimmune disease, which cause the immune system to attack healthy tissues of the body. Some examples are rheumatoid arthritis, lupus erythematosus, and multiple sclerosis. The connection between anxiety and free radicals is that when you have an excessive amount of anxiety, your body produces excessive amounts of a hormone called cortisol, which increases free radical production. There are also other pathways over which excessive anxiety has this effect.

The connection between emotional depression and immune system depression is that the immune system is really a circulating nervous system. When you feel emotionally depressed, the emotion results in the production of certain chemicals in the body called messenger molecules. The immune system responds to these messenger molecules just as the brain does. The immune system gets depressed. Then it is unable to do its usually competent job killing germs and cancer cells before they multiply enough to make you sick.

Knowing your answers to The Big Questions greatly reduces anxiety and makes you practically depression-proof as long as you are living, being, and doing what you know about yourself, your purpose, and your relationships to other people. There are many causes for anxiety, just as there are many branches on a big tree. Because of this, I like to find the root cause and get rid of that. I have had enough experience with trees to know that if I can cut the root, the branches are going to whither, die, and eventually disappear.

Regarding anxiety, I believe that the root cause is the knowledge that you are not fulfilling the purpose for which you came into this life. Dying with purpose unfulfilled is probably the worst thing that can happen. We believe that, on some level, everyone knows this. We also know that the clock is running. Every day we live brings the day of our death one day closer. The approach of death, and with it the ultimate horror of dying with purpose unfulfilled, is ample cause for fear. This process, operating outside conscious awareness, gives rise to anxiety. Anxiety feels like fear, but we do not know what we are afraid of. Some people call this existential anxiety, to contrast it with anxiety that comes from more superficial mental and emotional causes.

When anxiety hangs around too long, it is likely to turn into a form of depression. As with anxiety, there are many different causes of depression on the psychological and spiritual levels, but here again we are looking for the root cause. We believe that often it is despair of ever finding and fulfilling life's purpose. Finding out who you are makes it much easier for you to discover your purpose.

There is, of course, the other side of the coin. Once you know who you are, it gets easier to know your purpose for being in this life. Once you know what your purpose is, it becomes easier to understand the true nature of your relationship to the other people and things in your life. When you know why you are here and what to do with the people and things in your life, you have a choice to act to fulfill your purpose and create mutually beneficial, fulfilling relationships with people who are important to you. When you know that every day you are fulfilling some of your purpose, it is not so fearful to also know that every day brings your death a day closer. Carl's Granddaddy, about whom you will read in the Epilogue, went to his death as calmly as he went to dinner. He could do so because he had done everything he came into this life to do. Remember Justice Holmes' last words, "And now, the great adventure!"

As long as you are taking action every day to fulfill the purpose for which you came into this life, happiness comes into your life every day. Happiness is one of the most powerful antidotes to depression. If you feel enough happiness, you can not be depressed! Just as your body/mind makes certain kinds of messenger molecules when you are depressed, it makes other kinds when you are happy. When you are emotionally and spiritually happy, your immune system is also happy and goes whistling off into battle to lay waste to those first few germs or cancer cells before they can multiply enough to cause you trouble.

These are some of the mechanics by which anxiety and depression on one hand, and serenity and happiness on the other, decrease and increase your probability for the 100-year healthspan. We are not talking about a small increase or decrease either; we are talking about big differences—differences that can result in up to an 85% reduction in hospitalizations, for example.

There is another wonderful and powerful benefit from the discovery of your answer to "Who am I?" That is the experience of bliss. As wonderful and powerful as bliss is, we do not hear much about it. For one thing, it cannot be perceived by any of the five senses, so the superstition of materialism says it is not real or worth anything. A more important reason is that so few people experience it. Chopra defines bliss as a feeling of happiness that is not dependent on what happens. People feel happy when they get what the want—provided they really wanted what they thought they wanted. Bliss, on the other hand, is not dependent on what you get or do not get. It is the happiness that comes from being a conscious being, aware of living in a conscious, intelligent universe.

Bliss is a great blessing for several reasons. First, it just feels so good! Second, because it is not dependent on anything that happens or does not happen, nobody can take it away from you. Third, bliss helps you maintain balance in your life. You probably recall that balance is essential to activation of your self-healing mechanism, which you have to have in order to attain the 100-year healthspan and happiness along the way. The balancing power of bliss works like this: as long as you have a human body, you are going to have discomfort and stress. These will throw you out of balance if there is not a counterbalancing factor. Happiness will work as a counterbalance, but it is not dependable. It comes and goes according to circumstances that are not completely under your control. Bliss, on the other hand, is dependable. It is with you so long as you remember and be who you really are. In order to remember who you really are, you have to make that discovery in the first place. That is the point of this whole discussion. The part of you that experiences bliss is the highest part, your Higher Self. It is unlikely that you will be aware of it unless you know who you really are.

The clean rinse for the dirty-water brainwash

We have already considered how ignorance of your true nature creates vulnerability to manipulation and control by others. There are plenty of people who make careers of exploiting this vulnerability. Living under the control and exploitation of others is a miserable existence, totally incompatible with the 100-year healthspan.

The solution to this problem is to know and be your true self. Once you do that, you are in fact beautiful, powerful, effective, and happy. Once you have that experience within your own being and know it is not dependent on any other person, you are protected against manipulation whether it takes a form that sounds positive or negative. If this way of being sounds good to you, you may be interested in learning how to achieve it. We discuss that in the next two chapters.

HISTORICAL PERSPECTIVES

The main obstacle to knowing oneself is lack of direct experience of the highest aspect on one's Whole Self, the spirit, also known as the soul. The highest level of the spirit is Pure Consciousness. Since we already have some knowledge of all the other levels of ourselves, to be described in the next chapter, discovering true self, whom I call Whole Self, requires only gaining the experience of Higher Self. This is the ultimate key to answering the first big question, "Who am I?" Everything written here about the value of experiencing Pure Consciousness applies equally to discovering your self.

Appreciation of the value of the experience and application of the qualities of Pure Consciousness are nothing new. In fact, the spiritual practices of several of the great religions are designed to attain this level of consciousness. I believe it was this level of awareness and functioning, and the joy that results from it, that the Christ referenced when he said, according to Luke 17:21, "The Kingdom of God is within you." In Buddhism, there is this line from a Zen chant, "This earth where we stand is the Pure Lotus Land and this very body the body of Buddha." Each of the great religions prescribes a technology for attaining the strength of concentration and attention that permits awareness of Pure Consciousness. In Christianity, it is primarily prayer and various rituals.

In the Eastern religions, including Buddhism and Hinduism, it is meditation. Zen Buddhism probably has the best-developed technology that uses a variety of meditative paths to focus such intense attention on The Field of Pure Consciousness that one is able to perceive it with great clarity. The experience is called *satori*. Dyer writes about it in *Real Magic*. The best description I know of this experience of the sudden realization of this aspect of one's Whole Self, and the technology for attaining it, is in *The Three Pillars of Zen*, by Kapleau.

Richard Bucke, M.D., a Canadian psychiatrist, did a scientific study of this level of awareness and historical figures who have attained it and demonstrated its power. Bucke published his findings in *Cosmic Consciousness*. He concluded that such people as Muhammad, The Buddha, The Christ, Saint Paul, Shakespeare and Walt Whitman had achieved awareness of Pure Consciousness and had manifested its power in one way or another. Bucke wrote that, historically, only the most highly developed individuals, an infinitesimally tiny minority, ever gained this awareness of Pure Consciousness and access to its powers. He believed that humankind is now entering a stage in its evolution that will enable many people to do what only the greatest individuals of history attained.

James Redfield, in *The Celestine Prophecy* and several subsequent books, agrees with this position. The widespread interest in technologies for expanding awareness and in attaining higher states of consciousness suggests that Bucke and Redfield are correct. The ready access to mental and electronic technologies for strengthening the power of attention is part of this ultimately important and exciting process.

This book and the fact that you are reading it are further evidence for the accuracy of this perception. You are participating in the most powerful evolutionary leap in human history! This expansion of consciousness will correct a serious mistake in perception that has deprived millions of people of the quality and quantity of life they might have enjoyed. The misperception is that the experience of Pure Consciousness and the enjoyment of its qualities are accessible to human beings only after they had died and gone to heaven. Perhaps the Christ tried to correct this mistake when He said, "The Kingdom of Heaven is among you." If the scriptures are accurate, He did not say, "The Kingdom of Heaven will be among you after you die and go to heaven." He said, "The Kingdom of Heaven *is* among you." *Is* means now. We believe that what He said 2000 years ago was true then and is true now. The difference is that a significant fraction of humankind is now in the process of proving it for themselves — and for all humankind.

It is impossible to overestimate the importance of this process. It is the only way we know to solve problems and extinguish suffering that cannot be addressed from the level of consciousness at which the problems were created. It is a process that can only happen one person at a time. The only person you can make it happen to you is you, but once you do that, your seeing and being and doing will make it easier for others to do it for themselves. It is easier to walk through deep snow once the trail is broken, but each person must walk for himself or herself. The path is easier to travel at night when someone holds up a light, but each person must open his own eyes.

We have been considering the ultimate human achievement—and adventure. It depends on attaining the power of attention to maintain focus on The Field of Pure Consciousness sharply enough and long enough. This is not easy to do. For most people, it requires strong desire, determination, and consistent practice. We are, after all, considering a birthright of supreme value. It does not seem unreasonable that its acquisition and enjoyment would require strong effort and determination.

The hazards of passing a precious birthright on to a weak-willed and half-hearted heir, or even one who is not spiritually developed enough to use it wisely, has been demonstrated, particularly in cultures such as the British, in which primogeniture (giving the family fortune to the eldest son) was the custom. Many a magnificent birthright has been squandered and a noble family disgraced when the birthright passed into the hands of one lacking the self-discipline and insight to use it wisely. This may have been what the Nobel Laureate in Poetry, Rabindranath Tagore, had in mind when he wrote a poem to his Higher Power, expressing gratitude that access to Pure

Consciousness and its qualities was not easy, thus "...saving me from the peril of weak and uncertain desire."

One of the existentialist philosophers, I believe it was Kierkegaard, published an essay entitled "Purity of Heart Is To Desire One Thing." When the One Thing you desire is to know and be the qualities of Pure Consciousness, the desire will be fulfilled because you will do what is necessary to fulfill it. What is necessary is to gain and apply the power of concentration to keep attention focused on Pure Consciousness strongly enough and long enough. Doing so takes you through some remarkably austere terrain into an experience of unexcelled and unexpected splendor. The experience combines the excitement of high adventure, the ecstasy of love, and the blessing of bliss. It is a little like finally prying open an extraordinarily rough, tough, muddy oyster and finding an astonishingly large and lustrous pearl. In this case, the pearl is Pure Consciousness and its qualities. It is the ultimate source of everything, the ultimate refuge and the ultimate source of happiness. It is accessed through the mind-state of quiet alertness, the practice of meditation.

In spiritual life, even a sincere mistake taken seriously may have more value than halfhearted allegiance to theoretical or formal truth.

—Meher Baba

Chapter 7

WHO AM I? MEET YOUR WHOLE SELF!

"... that fierce joy that warriors feel in foemen worthy of their steel."

—Longfellow

INTRODUCTION

At the beginning of Chapter 6, we quoted Chopra: "Who am I? is the only question worth asking and the only one never answered." We consider that an unduly pessimistic conclusion. Most people may not be ready to invest the time, toil, and treasure necessary to find the full and final answer; but if they did, we believe they could.

For purposes of attaining your 100-year healthspan, finding the final answer is not necessary. A more modest attainment suffices: to be in the process of discovery and know enough of who you are to avoid the more dangerous dream destroyers and birthright burglars. For this, the discussion and directions in this chapter and the next will be useful.

In Chapter 6, we discussed five major obstacles to answering this First Big Question. There are specific tactical actions to overcome each of these obstacles. We present these interventions under the same headings we used in that chapter. You probably know which obstructions loom largest on your path. Your tactics will be wise if you use the countermeasures first that address those obstacles. If you do not know what to work on first, start with the Mistake of the Intellect. Tactically, that means meditation. In fact, anytime you do not know what to do next, meditation is probably your best choice. When you meditate, you access Pure Consciousness, where answers to all questions already exist. You may not find the answer right away, but you are looking in the right place.

While answering this first big question is strenuous and challenging, it will be worth far more than it costs. It is the adventure of a lifetime. The fun, fascination, and fulfillment of the quest are unequaled. The challenge is worthy of your best. Meeting it generates that fierce joy referenced at the beginning of this section. There is only one thing better: carried far enough, this process of discovery leads to the durable experience of bliss.

Since discovering who you are is the ultimate adventure, we suggest taking the same tactical approach that you would use if you were starting on a physical adventure. Suppose, for example, that your adventure includes crossing a wilderness to take possession of a priceless inheritance on the other side. Suppose that you knew the wilderness was rugged and vast, with five difficult and dangerous areas. Finally, suppose that you had a map and a guidebook. Before entering the wilderness, you would probably study the map and the guidebook carefully, and make sure you took them with you.

The ultimate adventure of self-discovery has each of these features. For most of us, the wilderness is ignorance of who we really are. The five dangerous and difficult areas are those we discussed in the preceding chapter: the condition of childhood, the brainwash with dirty water, the mistake of the intellect, the superstition of materialism, and sabotage by the ego. The diagram of The Whole Self, in the appendix, is the map—actually, a treasure map! Your Whole Self is the richest treasure in the universe. This chapter is a guidebook that tells you how to read the map. The next chapter tells how to cross each danger zone as safely and easily as possible. Now, let us study the map.

STUDY THE TREASURE MAP

Simply stated, you are your Whole Self. Your Whole Self is your domain, the rich, vast territory that you have inherited as your birthright. It is so vast that you have probably no more than caught a glimpse of it. It is so rich that you must explore it to believe it. The Whole Self Diagram is a small-scale map that can be a great help to you in your exploration. If you look at it frequently as you read this chapter and the next, you will gain more value in less time, with less headache risk.

My understanding of the structure and function of Whole Self is an integration of what I have learned from psychiatric training, from many years of psychiatric practice and spiritual practice, and from the works of Chopra and Meher Baba. Chopra's excellent audiotape album, *The Higher Self,* has been particularly helpful. Chopra's concept of Higher Self seems to come from Vedic teaching. For patients, students, and me the integration of ancient Vedic knowledge and wisdom with modern Western psychiatry and psychology has been remarkably powerful and useful. Most of our patients and students who have seen the diagram and heard the concept of the Whole Self in medical consultations, Healthspan Workshops, and seminars have been fascinated and have asked for copies of the diagram. Please consult it as we proceed.

The Whole Self consists of body, mind, and Higher Self. The Higher Self is also called the Spirit. We choose to use the former term because "Spirit" carries so much excess baggage of associations for many people that it may be a hindrance to understanding the Whole Self. With "Higher Self," a term most people have seldom or never heard, there is less likely to be preconceived notions and emotions that could obstruct understanding. Nobody is particularly surprised to hear that they have a body and a mind; but to some, the news that they also have a Higher Self is a novel and sometimes suspicious notion. This being so, let us start with the more familiar and proceed to the less so.

THE BODY: A MATTER OF MATTER AND ENERGY

I consider the body to have two basic components: matter and energy. Matter is well known scientifically and popularly. Its functions take place at the molecular level where biochemistry is the principal operational factor. The other component, energy, is more subtle. Chopra defines this energy as that which is necessary for all transformations that take place in the body-mind. For life to exist, transformations must go on continuously. It is estimated that between 4,000 and 5,000 chemical reactions go on constantly in the body. The food you eat has to be transformed into energy and into your own skin, muscles, blood, and bones. The thoughts you have must be transformed into neuropeptides and other messenger molecules so that your body can respond to your mind. The latent energy stored in certain molecules must be transformed into heat, electrical, and kinetic energy for your body-mind to function.

As powerful and essential to life as this subtle energy is, it cannot be perceived by any of the five senses, except after rigorous training or by extraordinarily perceptive people. There are very sensitive instruments capable of detecting some forms of subtle energy, such as that which radiates from the hands of healers. You may recall from the chapter The Power of Attention the discussion of some experiments on plants using this kind of energy.

Chinese medicine has recognized and manipulated this energy for millennia. Called *chi,* it is regulated by techniques including acupuncture, tai chi, chi gong and acupressure. In the West, these procedures have been incorporated into many natural healing systems in the last decade. By popular demand, they are beginning to be added to some systems of conventional medicine. A Western energy modulating procedure for healing is *therapeutic touch.* Touch has been used for healing throughout history, but was only recently brought into the field of scientific scrutiny and conventional medicine by the work of Delores Krieger, RN, and Ph.D.

We believe that we are at a historic transition point between healing paradigms in medicine. Biochemistry was the dominant paradigm in conventional medicine in the 20th century. Energy medicine, sometimes called vibrational medicine, will be the dominant paradigm of the 21st century—or at least an important part of the dominant paradigm. For a preview of how this may unfold, see *The Body Electric*, by Robert Becker, MD, *Vibrational Medicine*, by Richard Gerber, *Music Physician,* by Don Campbell, *Energy Anatomy*, by Caroline Myss, Ph.D. and the discussion in this book in Chapter 11: Balancing Energy.

The biochemical medicine of the 20th century was characterized by the development of antibiotics and the therapeutic use of hormones, particularly the adrenal steroids. Biochemical medicine was a great leap forward in dealing with infectious disease; but because it limited itself to the material level of the Whole Self, it was a great two-foot leap across a six-foot ditch, the other side of which is the 100-year healthspan. We now discover, to our dismay, that the ditch is full of water moccasins such as lethal, antibiotic-resistant bacteria, devastating side effects of steroids, and degenerative diseases such as rheumatoid arthritis, lupus erythematosus, and diabetes, for which conventional medicine has no definitive answer. Biochemical medicine has, at best, substantially reduced deaths from infectious disease and trauma and has "...enabled more of us to achieve senility."

Biochemical medicine is sometimes a good starting point for the leap to the 100-year healthspan—but it is only part of the leap. Of those who make only that part, the only ones who will be pleased with where they land will be those with an affinity for close encounters with water moccasins. Gaining the momentum necessary to land on the 100-year healthspan side of the ditch requires energy. Energy medicine and energy healing provide an important part of it.

In the 21st century, we will not discard biochemical medicine. We will use it for what it can do well and integrate it into a holistic system that will include energy medicine, mind medicine, and Higher Self medicine. If you want a jump-start on enjoying the benefits of 21st century medicine, you hold in your hands an instruction book on how-to.

THE MIND: EMOTION, INTELLECT, AND EGO

In this concept of The Whole Self, the mind has three components: emotions, intellect, and ego.

EMOTION: what changes thoughts to things.

Emotions are primarily feelings and desires. They guide the concepts and ideas developed by the intellect from the level of the intellect into the level of energy. This process is necessary for the transformations that result in an abstract idea manifesting as a material thing. For example, in the autumn, when the leaves begin to turn red, yellow, orange, and purple and the air gets cool, I get the idea that it would be good to cut some firewood. If there is no emotion associated with the idea, nothing gets added to the wood stack. But, if I enjoy cutting wood in the crisp, cool autumn air and thinking about a fire crackling cheerily in the soapstone stove on cold, snowy winter evenings, the emotion of enjoyment guides the idea from the level of intellect into the energy level of my body. Then the transformations take place that eventually lead to axe blade biting into wood and the woodstack starting to grow. Alternatively, if I do not enjoy cutting firewood, but fear being cold this winter when a blizzard takes out the power grid, that is another kind of feeling that can lead to the same result. Without emotion, the idea of splitting wood, and most other ideas, would probably come and fade away without any tangible trace.

INTELLECT: processing of ideas, beliefs and concepts to accomplish mission—or make mischief

The next level of mind is intellect. This is the function of the mind that manipulates ideas and beliefs into concepts that can be used as the blueprints for the creation of an infinite variety of things and events—this book, for example. A specialized function of the intellect is the ego, the aspect of intellect that contains the ideas, concepts, and beliefs that you have about yourself as a unique individual, separate from everyone else. Ego is the most powerful and important aspect of The Whole Self that we have yet considered. Its power comes from its ability to decide and control what ideas, beliefs, and concepts the intellect considers and which ones get the emotional charge they need for transformation into action.

EGO: a useful servant and a fearful master

Ego has so much power that it, like fire, makes a useful servant but a fearful master. If ego is under the control of the Higher Self, which we are about to consider, it makes key decisions about how we go about fulfilling our purpose in life. Uncontrolled from a higher level of Whole Self, ego is contentious, irritable, insatiably demanding, unreasonable, and always dissatisfied—in a word, egotistical. Ego gets a good bit of space in this book because it can be such a problem and a hazard to the 100-year healthspan. Now let us consider the level of the Whole Self and the technology from and by which ego can be controlled and mastered to become a wonderful servant.

THE HIGHER SELF: WHERE THINGS REALLY GET INTERESTING

Chopra conceptualizes the Higher Self as having two components: causal consciousness and Pure Consciousness.

CAUSAL CONSCIOUSNESS: "Whatever made me do that?!"

Causal consciousness is the repository of one's deepest and most powerful memories and desires. According to Vedic teaching, these memories and desires are so powerful that they carry over from one existence to the next. A growing body of scientific evidence indicates that this is actually happening. It certainly appeared to be happening in the case of the woman whose sudden recovery from disabling agoraphobia we described in

Chapter 4. The book, *Many Lives, Many Masters* by Brian Weiss, M.D., provides further support for this idea. Weiss presents a detailed case history of a patient who recovered from a serious emotional disorder as she recalled the experiences of several previous lifetimes. General George Patton is said to have believed that in a past life he had been Alexander The Great, and that his military genius was partly the memory of lessons learned and passion for victory remembered from his life as Alexander. Genevieve has a talent and love for music that appeared before she was five.

Wherever the memories and desires come from, they are so powerful that they shape thought and behavior, thus causing many of the experiences and events of one's life. The contents of causal consciousness are often outside of awareness, thus adding mystery to power. When someone says, "I can't imagine why I did that!" it may be that what he did was driven by some complex of memory and desire living in causal consciousness, but outside of awareness. Because these complexes are so powerful, it is better to be aware of them and to keep an eye on them, rather than getting blind-sided by them.

Chapter 5 presented the technology for expanding awareness into previously unconscious areas of causal consciousness. Sigmund Freud referred to this process in his famous statement about the goal of psychoanalysis: "And ego shall walk where Id was." To Freud, ego was awareness and Id was unconscious: i.e., outside awareness. Psychoanalysis has the ability to expand awareness into previously unconscious areas of the Whole Self, but in our experience, the use of the Quiet Alertness technology is more efficient, cost effective, and empowering for mission fulfillment.

As important as the repository function of causal consciousness is, it has another that is even more so. Chopra call it the "silent witness." From the section on "The Basis of Health" in Chapter 4, you may recall the discussion of the three aspects of awareness: the observer, what is observed, and the process of observation. The silent witness is the observer. If it is given enough attention, it can observe whatever you need to know. It can also make those observations without getting involved or entangled in anything it is observing—and it can experience bliss. In one of the Vedic texts, *The Mundaka Upanishad*, there is the statement, "Like two golden birds perched on the selfsame tree, the ego and the Self dwell in the same body. The former eats the sweet and sour fruits of life, while the latter looks on in detachment."

It is the ability of the silent witness to observe without involvement that makes it possible to control pain and suffering. My first experience of this came at a Zen meditation retreat, called *sesshin*. Sesshin requires sitting in meditation for several hours a day. I was new to meditation and very new to sitting in the lotus position for half an hour at a time, several times a day. Discipline in sesshin is strict: if one left the meditation room before meditation was over or moved too much, he might not be allowed to continue participation.

During a round of meditation, my hip started hurting. As the minutes passed the pain intensified, as though a fire were burning in my right hip joint. The slight movement permitted during meditation did not help at all. My impulse was to get up and leave the meditation room (*zendo*), but I was highly motivated to continue. I believed that Zen practice and participation in sesshin were the most direct route to fulfillment of a key part of my life mission, which was to discover the answer to the question "Who am I?" I was unwilling to jeopardize my access to the most direct route to enlightenment, but I could not stand the suffering.

In desperation, I remembered the advice of the Zen teacher on dealing with pain: put the attention in the center of the pain. Having no acceptable alternative, I did that with desperation-driven intensity. Within seconds, the pain began to diminish. In its place came the most intense experience of peace I had ever felt. My hip joint felt as though it had been numbed with a local anesthetic, but more astonishing was the wonderful experience of absolute peace and stillness. In amazement, I shifted my attention from the middle of where the pain used to be and put it on thinking about this incredible event. Instantly, the pain was back, worse than before, as though a red-hot spike were being driven into my hip joint. Back went my attention into the middle of the pain. Away went the pain. Back came the peace. I did not need another lesson.

Soon, the round of meditation was over. Everyone was free to stretch and walk around. I never again had severe pain while meditating. Although the experience occurred more than 20 years ago, I have never forgotten it—and never will.

That was my first experience of the power of putting all of my attention into the silent witness function of causal consciousness. With all attention there, other functions of awareness were suspended. Since the silent witness just observes without involvement in the scene, there could be no suffering, just awareness and peace. Viktor Frankl, M.D. used the power of the Silent Witness to survive in Nazi concentration camps.

As important as the capacity for awareness without suffering is, there is another function of the silent witness that is even more so. It is awareness of the highest and most wonderful level of Whole Self, called Pure Consciousness. In the ensuing discussion of Pure Consciousness, you may learn that there is more to your Whole Self than you ever imagined, and the *more* is more wonderful than you can imagine. In fact, were you unable to experience directly what we are about to write about, we probably would not even bother to do it because, if you have not already experienced it, you would never believe us. If you have already experienced it, you may be glad to know that two more people know it also. When everyone, or even a critical percentage of the population, has this experience of Pure Consciousness, there will be such a change in the relationships between people and their relationship to the earth that the quality of life for everyone on earth will improve. Sociologists say that the critical percentage is about 16. For evidence to support this contention, remember the section on "The Maharishi Effect" in Chapter 3.

Since the experience of Pure Consciousness is one of the greatest blessings for the individual and for the world, and since only the silent witness in Causal Consciousness can experience Pure Consciousness, you can begin to appreciate the value of this level and function of your Whole Self. Now let us consider the content and function of Pure Consciousness.

PURE CONSCIOUSNESS: THE MOST DELIGHTFUL SURPRISE

One of the greatest joys of writing this book is bringing incredibly good news—of a fabulous birthright unknown and unsuspected by most people. Nowhere is the news better than here, but we immediately encounter some major problems. One is that you may not take this knowledge seriously enough to investigate for yourself. That is a decision each person must make for self, so that is not our primary responsibility. Our responsibility is to bring the knowledge in the clearest, most attractive form and inspiring manner that we possibly can. The next problem is that the subject to be addressed lies beyond the reach of language. Human beings developed language to deal primarily with things and issues in the material world. Language serves that purpose and even can penetrate some distance into the nonmaterial dimensions, but for discussion of Pure Consciousness, language has severe limitations. So here is the dilemma: the most important knowledge must be brought in a vehicle grossly inadequate for the job. It is like trying to haul an elephant in a Honda Civic or carry the ocean in a wicker basket.

When I come to this part of a lecture or workshop, I take a deep breath, swallow hard, and go ahead. Now that I am writing this book, I do the same. I ask you to keep in mind that what you read will at best be a pale shadow of what you will experience when you energize your silent witness with the attention it must have to experience Pure Consciousness directly.

Pure Consciousness is shown in the diagram as the highest part of Whole Self because that is what it is: the most important and powerful aspect of Whole Self. Its qualities are humankind's most precious birthright, far more valuable than even the 100-year healthspan. In fact, these qualities must be recognized and manifested somewhat in order to attain the 100-year healthspan.

Here is a story of how two very different groups of people came to similar conclusions about what these qualities are. One group consisted of quantum physicists: scientists who study the ultimate source of the universe and the way something comes out of nothing. This group is on the cutting edge of modern science. Quantum physicists study the boundary between energy and matter where the transition occurs between energy and sub-atomic particles, and vice versa. On one side of this boundary is the material universe; on the other side is the nothingness out of which the universe emerges. They call this nothingness "The Unified Field."

The other group consists of Vedic scholars: students and practitioners of the most ancient wisdom system on record, The Vedas. The Vedas have their own version of how the universe came into existence and what its source is. They call this Source "Pure Consciousness." Quantum physicists and Vedic scholars do not usually talk to one another, so nobody knew how their views compared until Maharishi Mahesh Yogi asked some Quantum physicists to list the qualities of the Unified Field and some Vedic scholars to list the qualities of Pure Consciousness. It may have occurred to the Maharishi to do this because he is trained both as a Vedic scholar and a physicist.

When the lists were compared, the qualities were identical. What a remarkable thing! The oldest and the newest knowledge systems agree on the qualities of the ultimate source of the universe. It does not matter whether this source is called The Unified Field or Pure Consciousness: the qualities are the same. I call it Pure Consciousness because that is the way I experience it and that is the way it makes the most sense to our students and patients.

Here is a list of those qualities. They may be of interest to you for reasons just mentioned and because they are the qualities of the highest part of your Whole Self. That makes them your qualities, part of your birthright, which you may want to claim and use. One of my instructors in ayurvedic physician's training gave me the list. I subsequently saw it in material Chopra distributed at one of his seminars. It is reproduced here with his kind permission.

Here is the list:
  Total potential of natural law
  Infinite organizing power
  Fully awake within itself
  Infinite correlation
  Perfect orderliness
  Infinite dynamism
  Infinite creativity
  Pure knowledge
  Unboundedness
  Perfect balance
  Self-sufficiency
  All possibilities
  Infinite silence
  Harmonizing
  Evolutionary
  Self-referral
  Invincibility
  Immortality
  Unmanifest
  Nourishing
  Integrating
  Simplicity
  Purifying

Freedom

Bliss

Quite a list! It will raise some questions. What do some of these strange terms mean? If these really are the qualities of Pure Consciousness, a part of my Higher Self that is part of my Whole Self, why do I not experience these qualities in the details of my daily life? If I do not experience these qualities and I want to experience, use, and enjoy them, how do I do that? We will answer these questions in the next chapter, in the section on the clean rinse after the dirty-water brainwash.

Chapter 8

WHO AM I? The PROCESS of DISCOVERY

INTRODUCTION

In the previous chapter, we began to get acquainted with the map of the Whole Self. Are you beginning to get the idea that this territory might be bigger, more complex, and more magical than you imagined? Feeling a little excited and eager to start exploring it? If so, before you go, take time to learn how to cross the tricky places. Bob Dylan sang, "Gonna know my song well before I start singin'." That is an excellent precept for this adventure. Some of the places you have to traverse are difficult—and dangerous, too, in the sense that if you do not know what to do, you can get so lost and confused that you give up and lose out. There is also the risk of making yourself and others unnecessarily uncomfortable while you are crossing the hazardous areas, if you do not know how to do it skillfully. Any adventure carries these risks—otherwise, it would not be an adventure. The prudent approach is to learn as much as you can before you begin, then pay moment-by-moment attention to what is happening as the adventure unfolds. Now, let us consider the problem areas in the order in which they occur; first is the condition of childhood.

CORRECTING THE CONDITION OF CHILDHOOD

Adaptation

One of the biggest dangers here is that you will spend so much of your time and energy adapting to and trying to please others that you will not have enough left to finance your adventure. How about an evaluation of your adaptation budget? One simple but useful way to get answers to how much time and energy you spend each day trying to live up to what you *think* other's expectations are, is to spend some time each night before going to bed, thinking about the events of the day. How many times did you make decisions based on what you believed would be right and best? When, during the day, did you make decisions based on trying to please others? Genevieve did this experiment during a year's clinical training in Transactional Analysis. She found that she spent at least 90% of her time and energy each day thinking about what the neighbors or friends or family would think, and what the children and I wanted her to do.

Only when you experience what an energy drain it is to try to please others, are you ready to direct more energy into discovering the real you that you lost in the situation of childhood, and getting in contact with what *you* want and need to do with your life.

Basic human needs

A useful aspect of getting back in contact with the real you is to become aware of what your physical, spiritual and emotional needs are. When Genevieve has asked her counseling clients what their needs are, they have usually been able to come up with food, rest, and protection from the elements. That is a good start, but it is far from complete. A list of basic human needs may be helpful:

- Recognition (Having someone speak your name or say "Hello". This basic need is why we use time out with children and solitary confinement with criminals.)

- Sensuality (To be aware of and experience all senses. Since the skin is the largest sense organ in the body, we need to be touched regularly in a loving way. Transactional Analysis says that if we do not get enough hugs, our spinal cord shrivels up!)

- Nutritious food

- Pure, clean air

- Pure water

- Regular physical exercise

- Regular contact with Mother Earth

- Proper rest and adequate sleep

- Intimacy (emotional; sexual intimacy is considered a "hunger," not a need.)

- Intellectual stimulation

- Fun and laughter

- Spontaneity

- Quiet time alone (meditation)

- Loving and being loved

- Being creative

- Being in the process of discovering and being my true self

- Finding my purpose in life and being in the process of fulfilling that purpose

- Living mindfully (giving full attention to what is going on right now, rather than remembering the past or imagining the future)

- Experiencing and cultivating a relationship with a Higher Power (call it God, Higher Consciousness, The Supreme Being, whatever. What you call this Power is not important; that you experience a Higher Power is all-important.)

- Forgiving and being forgiven

In addition to the above, each of us has needs unique to us. For instance, Genevieve needs to listen to and participate regularly in some musical experience. Cooking nutritious foods is one of her creative needs. She also enjoys eating what she has prepared! So, do I, who consider my enjoyment, day-in and day-out, of delicious, wholesome food to be one of the blessings of my life.

Unfortunately, people define themselves by the roles they play. It is helpful to write down what roles you play and to become aware of the time and energy you spend fulfilling them. Then, you may wish to decide how much time and energy you will redirect to taking care of your needs, one of the most important of which is fulfilling the purpose for which you came into this world.

THE CLEAN RINSE AFTER THE DIRTY WATER BRAINWASH

The brainwash starts in childhood, but does not stop there. All your life, you meet people who will tell you whatever they think will induce you to do what they want you to do. Some of this will be about who you are—not that they care who you are, or have a clue about it. Some people are effective manipulators because they have discovered that many people are either hungry to know who they are or terrified to find out; so misinformation or disinformation disguised as information on the subject is particularly effective for manipulation. Since this is a hazard you can expect to be meeting all your life, you might as well have an effective way to deal with it.

The wisest and most powerful level of your Whole Self is Pure Consciousness. That makes it the ideal level from which to deal with attempts to manipulate you. Unfortunately, the Higher Self level is also the least familiar. One of life's ironies is that what is most important to us is least known and used. You may recall from your map study a few pages ago that one of the qualities of Pure Consciousness is pure knowledge. This includes knowing who you are. We suggest beginning to experience and use this quality, together with some of the others that interest you. We will now tell you how. Together, they will provide a powerful clean rinse after the brainwash.

It is time to address the question, "If these really are the qualities of Pure Consciousness, which is part of my Whole Self, why don't I experience them in the details of my daily life?" To respond to the natural doubt about possessing qualities of great value that you have never experienced, we will say that if we did not know that you *could* experience them, we would not bother to write about them. When something sounds preposterous, the only way we know to believe it is to experience it. Here is how to do it: *use the power of attention.*

Even after writing a long chapter on "The Power of Attention," we have understated the case. In simple terms, where you put and hold your attention determines whether or not you experience, use, and enjoy these qualities of Pure Consciousness in your daily life. Where you put and hold your attention determines whether or not you experience the ultimate adventure of discovering and fulfilling your mission in this life. In fact, attention is so powerful that it is dangerous to let it stay on anything you do not wish to expand in your life. Like a sharp blade or a power saw, it is dangerous when used carelessly. However, used skillfully, attention, like sharp, powerful tools, will enable you to build joyfully what would otherwise be difficult or impossible.

Skillful, persistent focusing of attention will enable you to experience directly the qualities of Pure Consciousness. You may wish to review the list at the end of the preceding chapter.

Focusing attention on an abstract quality like "freedom" or "perfect orderliness" is hard work. If you need more motivation to do this work—and directly experience these qualities that are already yours—it may help to understand some of the mechanics by which attention brings abstract qualities into action. Action then produces tangible results in your life. An excellent discussion of this is in Chopra's *Creating Affluence*. In Chapter 3: "The Magic of Attention," he uses some principles of quantum physics to illustrate the process.

Quantum physics explores the border between the Unified Field and the material universe. On the Unified Field side of the border, there is intelligence and energy, but no thing—nothing material. Just across the border, on the material universe side, there are subatomic particles. They have names like quarks, leptons, and bosons, but the important thing about them is that they are the smallest and most basic building blocks of atoms, which are the building blocks of the entire material universe. These subatomic particles are constantly appearing on the material universe side of the border and disappearing on the Unified Field side. Something powerful, mysterious, and magical is happening on that border. Something is making material things appear and disappear out of intelligence and energy. That *something* is attention!

Quantum physicists have discovered that every subatomic particle is a wave at the same time. A wave is energy; it is not a material thing. It exists everywhere as the *possibility* of turning into a material thing. What actually causes the transformation? Attention! When attention is focused on the Unified Field, waves turn into subatomic particles—i.e., they cross the border, and *energy* becomes a *thing*. When attention is withdrawn, turned elsewhere, the particle goes back across the border and becomes energy again. It disappears and no longer even exists. There is only the possibility that it will exist again through the magic of someone's attention. Here modern science presents some of the mechanics of a process described by the Buddha 2,500 years ago: "With our thoughts we make the world."

What does all this have to do with your experiencing qualities of your Higher Self? Before you focus your attention on these qualities, they are like the wave on the Unified Field side of the border. They exist as *possibilities* that you will experience, use, and enjoy, but they are just possibilities. To cross the border and become real, active parts of your Whole Self, they have to have your attention, just as waves of energy in the Unified Field have to have someone's attention to turn into material particles. So, the crucial question becomes, "If I want to experience and use these qualities in the details of my daily life, how do I give them my attention?" Chopra suggests two methods. I have validated them personally and clinically. They work!

The first is to put your attention on a quality of Pure Consciousness and hold it there. That sounds simple enough, but it is hard to do, and *how* you do it makes a critical difference. The hard part you can overcome with practice of the skills you read about in Chapter 4. There is more about building your power of attention in the section on "The Flick Protocol" in Chapter 11.

Now, here is how to do it skillfully. Select one quality of Pure Consciousness for each day of the month. For example, suppose that for today you selected "perfect balance." Today, hold those words in your awareness by focusing your attention on them. Do it the same way you would focus attention on a phone number you want to remember until you can write it down. You do not try to interpret the number, or define it, or analyze it. You just focus attention on it so that it stays in your awareness. That is exactly what you do with "perfect balance." You do not try to interpret the words or the concept or try to analyze them or define them; you just keep your attention focused on the words whenever your attention does not need to be focused on something else. The main magic of doing this is that the quality of perfect balance grows stronger in your life. You find yourself doing things you would not ordinarily do that result in your life coming into better balance. It is like the quantum physicist focusing attention on the Unified Field. The wave becomes the particle. For you, the magic is that the *possibility* of perfect balance becomes *movement toward* perfect balance in your life—an actual improvement in balance on one or more levels of your Whole Self. For example, when you need to balance indoor time with more outdoor time, you may be surprised at how easy it is to switch off the TV and go out for a walk. When you need to balance social activity with solitude, you may find yourself choosing to meditate more and socialize less, even though you had not made that choice before.

Most people are not going to spend all day focusing attention on some quality of Pure Consciousness. If they did, they would probably experience things so powerful that they would be called miraculous, but life is not structured to favor spending a day that way. Even if it were, most people do not have such powerful control over where they put their attention. Since, in real life and real time, attention is going to be on many other things during a day, how can this process work? You can make it work by putting your attention on the quality-of-the-day when attention does not need to be on something else. For example, you do it when you are holding a phone that someone has put on hold, or when you are sitting in a traffic jam and cannot move. More importantly, you do it when your attention perversely focuses on something you definitely do not want expanding in your life, like getting Alzheimer's or getting mugged.

Many people have thoughts that they find disturbing, but cannot put out of their minds. Obsessive-compulsive disorder (OCD) is an extreme form of this problem. It is possible to put such thoughts to work for you by letting them remind you to put your attention on the Quality of the Day. You can create an association between the bothersome thought and returning your attention to the Quality of the Day by thinking, "Well! Here is that bothersome thought again. It is time to put my attention back on the Quality of the Day."

Wayne Dyer is right: the only thing over which we have complete control is what we think. A person who has OCD may not believe that he has control over what he thinks, but he can gain that control through increasing the power of attention. The process is often easier if he is using one of the drugs or amino acids that increase the action of serotonin in the nervous system.

If you watch much TV, a wonderful option would be to watch a little less and spend the redeemed time focusing on the quality-of-the-day. You could even mute the commercials and have time to increase perfect balance in your life. Most people spend more time than they like putting attention on things that make them upset or sick. You can train yourself to make that a signal to focus on the quality-of-the-day.

Since I tend to forget to do this, I write the quality-of-the-day in red at the top of the page of the day in my Franklin Covey Planner. You will read about that aid for mission fulfillment and happiness in the chapter, "Why Am I Here?" Since I look at that page frequently, I get reminded to use this technique for bringing one of the qualities of Pure Consciousness into action in my life.

The second way Chopra recommends experiencing the qualities of Pure Consciousness is to put your attention into the Field of Pure Consciousness. When you do this, instead of focusing on one quality, you become aware of them all at once. Of course, no particular one is so clear and vivid as when you focus on it alone, but being able to experience the whole picture at once is at least as valuable as seeing each quality clearly and in detail. As you probably know by now, you put your attention into the Field of Pure Consciousness by creating the mind-state of quiet alertness, using one of the paths Genevieve wrote about in Chapter 5. When you do this, you not only become aware of the sum total of all the qualities of Pure Consciousness, but you also either activate these qualities in your life all at once or automatically select the ones you need most. In any case, when you experience Pure Consciousness, it is the most wonderful experience you are ever likely to have. One thing that makes it so is that you become aware of these qualities —a rich and wondrous legacy that you probably had no idea belonged to you.

Most people do not experience this all at once; most of us gain the experience a little at a time over a period of years. The neurofeedback technology mentioned in Chapter 5 can shorten that time by years, but, for most people, it still is not going to happen all at once. The important thing is that you do not have to have the whole, clear experience in order to feel better, function better, and experience the delicious excitement of knowing that there is powerful magic here. The improvement in feeling and functioning starts as soon as you get the first glimpse, and maybe even before. It may start the first time you do the quiet alertness technology, although the experience may be so subtle you hardly notice it.

This whole technology for realizing the qualities of Pure Consciousness in your life is so powerful and so important that it would be worth your while to read about it from Chopra's perspective in *Creating Affluence*. By combining what you learn from each source, you will probably have a more effective system to work for you—better than what you could get from either one alone.

By the time you have waded through this long, abstract although critically important discussion, we think you deserve to hear how this can be valuable in real life. One example is this book. Had we not used this technology, accessed some of these qualities, and let them work in the writing process, you would not be reading this now.

What are the mechanics? Let us start with the first quality, Total Potential of Natural Law. Natural Law refers to all the laws of nature. These are the laws that uphold the integrity of the universe and govern the creation of everything that comes into existence. Natural law is the source of everything that has ever existed and everything that now exists. Natural law has the potential to create an unlimited range of things and events that have never before existed. The total potential of natural law underlies the quality of Pure Consciousness that is called All Possibilities. Had we not known these qualities of Higher Self through direct experience, we would not have started this book because we would not have believed we could complete it.

Some other qualities came in handy, too. Infinite Organizing Power was essential to the organization of a mass of data that at first was chaos. Perfect Orderliness brought some order, obviously not perfect, out of the chaos. Infinite Dynamism supplied the sustained, intense energy necessary to bring *Healthspan* into form while serving a medical practice, evolving our spiritual practices, maintaining some semblance of balance and harmony in our Whole Selves, and filling the roles we have chosen for ourselves: father, mother, sister, teacher, and friend. In this complex balancing process, Infinite Correlation was essential. So was Perfect Balance. As we write "Perfect," we are perfectly aware that none of what we have done is perfect. The perfection exists in our Higher Selves, in Pure Consciousness, as it does in yours and everyone else's. However, that does not mean that the perfection manifests in what we do—this book or anything else. This is partly because our attention is not perfectly focused in Pure Consciousness and because we allow Causal Consciousness and Ego to obstruct and distort the perfection of the outflow from Pure Consciousness. We work every day to reduce the obstruction and distortion. It is decreasing, but there is clearly more work to be done.

Some other qualities that were vital to the production and mission fulfillment of *Healthspan* are Evolutionary, Nourishing, Simplicity (we wish there were more of that; we bet you do, too), Purifying, and Freedom. If this book does not possess these qualities and does not to some degree transmit them to you, it cannot fulfill its mission to be of assistance in the healing of injury and disease, the cessation of suffering, and the attainment of full enlightenment and your 100-year healthspan.

ACCEPT NO LIMITATIONS!

There is not a man alive who cannot do more than he thinks he can.

—Henry Ford

One ingredient in the brainwash is conditioning to doubt and grossly underestimate your abilities. After all, people who want to control you need for you to need them. They are not likely to encourage you do develop your abilities and self-sufficiency. Therefore, over the years, most people fall farther and farther behind in fulfilling their potential for attainment in practically every area.

Dyer has an antidote for the poison of self-doubt. In *Real Magic,* he wrote, "Accept no limitations." Earlier, I mentioned quoting him to the neurologist who criticized me for presenting the 100-year healthspan as a possibility. Since the concept is important, I will expand it here. Dr. Dyer's reasoning for this seemingly unreasonable suggestion is that no one knows what he can do until he tries it. As soon as one accepts a limitation, he is bound by it. Remember Stephen Covey saying, "Argue for your limitations and they are yours!" Once you know from your own direct experience that in the Field of Pure Consciousness there is the total potential of natural law, thus making it the field of all possibilities, Dyer's advice becomes entirely reasonable and wonderfully wise.

The lives of some of my patients may depend on my ability to communicate this to them. I have a "resort practice": some of my patients come to me as a last resort. The first time this happened, many years ago in Albany, Georgia, a disheveled, distraught man came into my consulting room. He said he had been on his way to the Flint River to commit suicide by jumping off the bridge. While on the way, he recalled that someone had told him we did weird things at The Wellness Center. He thought that whatever we did was probably not so weird as jumping off the Flint River bridge, so he swung by to see if I had a better idea. He eventually agreed that I did; he went on to apply a less destructive solution to his problems.

Since that time, more and more "last resort" patients have consulted me. Some of them, like Ken, mentioned in Chapter 1, have been under a medical death sentence. Others, who have chronic conditions that are not likely to be fatal (except to their quality of life), have been told that nothing can be done for them and they have to "learn to live with it." I sometimes suggest to those patients that they "Learn to live without it." I may then go on to say that when they put their attention in The Field of Pure Consciousness, they are positioning themselves for a miracle healing. I do not guarantee that it will happen, but I mention that if you want to get struck by lightening during a thunderstorm, your chances are better standing on the roof holding a golf club overhead than if you are in the basement sitting on a stack of tires. Of course, I do much more than that, but I do point out that the more the attention is focused in Pure Consciousness the better the prognosis is and the better all the other things I prescribe are going to work. That is because attention brings qualities, including infinite correlation, perfect orderliness, infinite dynamism, perfect balance, all possibilities, nourishing, purifying, and bliss, from the *possibility* that they *might* appear or increase to *actual manifestation* in the patient's life.

After a few experiences of succeeding in doing things you thought you could not do, the dirty water starts rinsing away. By using Chopra's protocol, you discovered that you possess qualities nobody ever told you that you had. By taking Dyer's prescription, you put some of those qualities to work. The result rinsed out some of the brainwash. Can you see how this can get to be fun?

SHEDDING THE SUPERSTITION OF MATERIALISM

The same things we have just considered for rinsing out the brainwash help with the superstition, but one more part needs to be added. It is an experiment to test the validity of the superstition. You can do a test to see if it is really true that the only things that have reality and value are those that you can see, hear, taste, touch, and/or smell. Here is how.

Think of some thing that you crave but do not have. Make it something that you can detect with one or more of your five senses. For one month, work as hard as you can to get it. If you succeed, enjoy it to the fullest. For the next month, select the quality of Pure Consciousness that you would most like to have more of in your life. Spend the month working as hard as you can, using Dr. Chopra's procedures, to manifest that quality in your life. At the end of the month, consider which has brought you more pleasure, peace, and power: the thing you desired and worked to get, or the quality of Pure Consciousness that you focused your attention on. If you did not get the thing or fully manifest the quality, which effort brought more value into your life?

It really makes less difference than you might think whether you got the thing you were trying for. You have probably noticed that no *thing* brings the pleasure, joy, and contentment you expected—at least, not for long. Now you know why: ego has incurable "more" disease. Ego is like the land-hungry farmer who said, "I'm not greedy. I just want what j'ines mine." No matter how much of a thing you get, ego wants more and is chronically dissatisfied. Fortunately, ego has no interest in the qualities of Pure Consciousness; ego does not want them in the first place, and certainly does not want more of them. It just ignores them and so its dissatisfaction does not spoil your enjoyment.

When you notice more value coming into your life from spending your time and energy on manifesting a quality than on getting a thing, you begin to question the superstition. That is the first step toward breaking it. Once you break it, or even weaken it, your progress toward answering the First Big Question accelerates.

Genevieve has had some experience with this process. Let her tell you about some of them.

"In October of each year while our children were at home, we took them out of school and went to the mountains for a week to camp, hike, and enjoy the fall color. One year we pitched our tents on an island in the Oconaluftee River at Mr. Owl's Campground. Every moment while we were in camp we could hear the sound of the water as it rushed by our island. The children spent happy hours skipping stones across the river while I prepared our meals. On the third night, after watching two complete cycles of the sun going down in the west and rising in the east, I awoke about 4:00 the next morning to a beautiful moonlit sky. Everything was still and quiet except for the sound of the river. I was flooded with a sense of awe, peace and contentment such as I had never known before. This experience came during a time in my life when I was still pushing myself unmercifully, trying to get perfect enough at *something* so that my father would approve of me. For a time, I was totally one with my Mother Earth; I felt my heart beating regularly with the heartbeat of the earth. The significance of this event was that it crystallized in my mind the understanding that I did not have to be stressed out and trying for perfection all the time; peace was now a possibility that I could experience—if I could just find the way.

"The second time that I had an experience of higher consciousness occurred when I was invited to play the organ at a large church while the organist was recovering from surgery. I had minored in organ in college but had burned myself out with music and had been "retired" for 25 years. The first Sunday morning that I was to play, I arrived at the church at 7:30 a.m. to get my fingers and feet accustomed to playing that beautiful, huge pipe organ before time for the 8:30 service that was televised to all of south Georgia. Only the janitor and TV crews were there.

"I tried to play, but my hands and legs were shaking so uncontrollably that I knew that I could not play with that much stage fright. What to do? I closed my eyes and visualized a hole in the top of my head with God's love pouring through my head and into my heart, arms, hands, legs, and feet. I held this vision in my mind until I was calm. When I opened my eyes, the choir had assembled and was ready to start practicing for the service. No, I did not cover myself with glory or play perfectly, but I didn't miss any cues and I didn't play any bad notes. I became "one" with the organ, the music, and the congregation. I finished playing the postlude for the 11:00 o'clock service and sat down to take off my organ shoes. I knew that I had won a battle with stage fright that had plagued me every time I had played in public, beginning with my first piano recital when I was five years old.

"One evening a friend called to say that his wife had died that day from an incurable, chronic illness and that she had requested that I play the piano at her funeral. I insisted that I did not have the time to get my fingers limber enough to play the piano on such short notice, but he would not take no for an answer. He gave me the names of the songs she had requested, some of which were organ/piano duets that I had never played. I spent what little practice time I had learning the duets, instead of practicing to limber my fingers. I would do the best I could, period. After the organist and I had played the pieces we did together, I played the hymns that my friend had requested, but I miscalculated the timing somehow and had time left before the family came in. Without skipping a beat, music began flowing from my fingers—melodies I had never heard! My fingers were not stiff; they seemed to caress each key gently as the music filled the church. I did not play the piano; my fingers seemed to be controlled by something outside me, yet deep within me."

Each of these experiences further weakened the grip of the superstition of materialism, giving Genevieve more freedom to discover and be who she is. Similar adventures await you!

When you first begin to experience these qualities of Pure Consciousness, they may not seem to make much difference in your life. This is partly because you get only fleeting glimpses of them before your attention wanders back to its usual territory. Remember the subatomic particle disappearing back across the quantum border as soon as attention is directed away from the Unified Field? The same thing happens to the quality of Pure Consciousness when attention is directed elsewhere. When your power of attention is strong enough to keep attention on Pure Consciousness for longer intervals, you will feel the power of its qualities grow stronger and see more evidence of their activity in your life. They are part of your birthright, a major source of happiness, wonder, joy, and real magic. They are necessary for the experience of mental, physical, and social well-being until you are 100 years old or more. The sooner you experience them and put them to work for you, the better. I know of nothing else that approaches their power to "add years to your life and life to your years."

CORRECTING THE MISTAKE OF THE INTELLECT

The mistake of the intellect is awareness of all the things, thoughts and people in one's life without the counterbalancing, simultaneous awareness of the Unity from which they all came, and to which they will all return. Ayurveda maintains that the mistake of the intellect is the basis of disease. I maintain that ayurveda is right. For a review of this pivotal concept, see the section on *The Basis of Health* in Chapter 4.

The mistake of the intellect is the root cause not only of disease but also of ignorance of who one really is. As long as the intellect is aware only of diversity, it cannot be aware of Pure Consciousness, which includes the unified basis of everything.

Until you are aware of Pure Consciousness, you can never know who you are. That is another reason that the mistake of the intellect is deadly to your chances for the 100-year healthspan or any durable happiness. Fortunately, the mistake is correctable. You can review the technology for correction in the above referenced section in Chapter 4. Since the mistake is corrected by meditation, which has a uniquely broad spectrum of additional benefits, it is wise to give meditation top priority in the adventure of finding your answer to the First Big Question.

SABOTAGE BY THE EGO: SABOTAGING THE SABOTEUR

Oh God, Grant me the wisdom to know Your will,
the strength and the courage to do it,
and the grace to do it in a way that pleases You.
Amen.

—OJW

Ego makes endless trouble because of its incurable "More" disease. It can never be satisfied or contented because it is built on the mistake of the intellect, not on the reality of the oneness of all life. It always feels its falseness and emptiness; it always persists in the futile, frustrating fight to get more and more things to fill the emptiness. Since it always fails in that attempt, it is always angry. The anger poisons the wellspring of life. This makes ego a major hazard to the 100-year healthspan. Getting rid of it is one of the most powerful things you can do to claim your birthright—and also one of the most difficult. Ego has great power because it controls which of your deep unconscious desires and memories get access to your intellect. Ego is like the computer "Hal", in"2001: A Space Odyssey". The computer was created to serve the crew of the space ship, but took on a will and a life of its own and began to kill the crew to protect itself when the crew tried to shut it down.

Ego will do its best to sabotage all efforts to reduce its power and control over your life. It is invulnerable to frontal assault, but you can sabotage this wily saboteur. Here is an adaptation of a method described by Meher Baba:

1. Focus your attention on your Higher Power. Make your Higher Power the object of your meditation. After meditation, maintain that focus of attention as much of the time as possible. When you awaken each morning, immediately establish that focus of attention. Return to it again and again throughout the day. Let any strong emotion or intense experience remind you. Use boredom as a reminder, too. After you go to bed at night, hold that focus as consciousness fades into sleep.

2. Cultivate intense love for your Higher Power. Your love may flow spontaneously as you become increasingly aware of the beauty, grace, blessings, and divine love constantly flowing from your Higher Power to you. The greater your power of attention, the more of this awareness you have.

If your love for your Higher Power does not readily come into your awareness and grow stronger, there are some things you can do to nurture it. Cultivating the attitude of gratitude is one of them. If you wish to use this, review Genevieve's discussion in Chapter 5. Another way is to recall the most loving relationship or experience you can remember. As you do this, a feeling will come into your awareness that is the emotional signature of that loving experience. Hold that feeling in your awareness. Now include your Higher Power in your awareness. Hold both in your awareness as long and as strongly as possible. In this way, you will develop an association between awareness of your Higher Power and the experience of deep, powerful love. Once the association is established, it will grow stronger as the magic of your relationship evolves.

There is a way to combine this procedure with a chi gong practice, which I will describe in Chapter 13. Most people like two-for-the-price-of-one sales. This combination is the ultimate: two important benefits in the same amount of time it takes to get one—plus powerful synergy.

3. The feeling of intense love produces a strong desire to please the one toward whom you feel love. Through sustained power of attention on your Higher Power, you learn what your Higher Power wants you to do in each situation you encounter. When knowing what to do meets strong desire to do it, action is likely. That action probably will not please ego. Ego will try to sabotage it, but love is the one force against which ego cannot prevail. If your love is strong enough, you will override ego—and take a step toward making it your servant instead of your master.

4. Once you have completed the action, offer it as a gift to your Higher Power, forget that you did it, and go on to the next situation that needs your attention. If you cannot forget it completely, think, "My Higher Power did that through me; I was only the agent." Avoid thinking, "I did that."

5. Each time you use this sequence, your love for your Higher Power becomes stronger and ego becomes weaker. It may not always feel that way, because ego will fight harder at times than others. You will not win every battle, but if you persist, you will

win the war. When you win the war, you have removed an absolute obstacle to discovering who you really are.

In this way, you can gradually make the transition from responding to orders from your ego to responding to your Higher Power. This will short circuit and sabotage your ego. Deprived of your attention, which is its source of energy, it will gradually weaken, losing its power to delay your progress toward discovering who you really are.

In this process, you will gradually transfer control of your life from your ego to your Higher Power. As you do so, you will enter what Chopra calls the zone of spontaneous right action. In that zone, you know the appropriate thing to do at the appropriate time. As you live and act in this zone, harmony replaces conflict, love replaces fear, order replaces chaos, contentment replaces anger, fulfillment replaces frustration, and happiness replaces suffering. This process is one of the most important things you will ever do to claim and enjoy your birthright.

CONCLUSION

We have now considered five of the dangerous areas you need to negotiate on the way do answering the First Big Question. You have gained knowledge of how to deal with each of them. As you progress on your adventure, you may wish to refer to this chapter several times. We wish you a safe and triumphant journey!

Whether you say "I can" or "I can't," you are right.

—Henry Ford

Chapter 9

WHY AM I HERE? THE POWER of PURPOSE

So long as you have a why,
you can make do with almost any how.

—Nietzsche

JAILBREAK!

In *Real Magic*, Dyer writes about the importance of being "on purpose." When I was treating Leroy at the mental health center, I had a good opportunity to see what Dyer meant. Leroy had been plagued with recurrent major depression and post-traumatic stress disorder since he served in the Army in Vietnam in the seventies. For the past twenty years, he had been in and out of VA hospitals for treatment of those conditions. The treatments had not given him much relief. When he was not in the hospital, he was dealing cocaine. He had gotten caught, tried, convicted and sentenced to long time.

When I first saw him he was severely depressed and looked like death. As he described his life to me, it was clear that it had been, and still was, a living hell. I did what I could for him with brief interviews and antidepressant medication, but we kept running into the limitations imposed by Dr. Sidney Baker's First Tacks Law: "When you are sitting on a tack it takes a lot of Elavil to make that feel good." In Leroy's case, when he was sitting in jail looking back on twenty years of unrelieved desolation and devastation and looking forward to another twenty in prison, it really was going to take a lot of Elavil to make that feel good.

Since Leroy looked ready; that is, desperate enough to try almost anything, I said to him, "Leroy, it doesn't look like you're going to be able to get your body out of jail right now, but would you be interested in getting your mind out?"

At that point, the prospect of getting anything of his out of jail was attractive to Leroy. I had his attention. I reached in the desk, pulled out a copy of *Real Magic*, held it where he could see it and said, "In this book there are detailed instructions about how you can get your mind out of jail." Then, I handed the book to him. He looked skeptical, puzzled, and hopeful at the same time. He left with the book.

Two weeks later a deputy sheriff brought Leroy in again. This time he did not look quite so depressed. He said, "Doc, that's a good book." I asked him if he noticed what Dr. Dyer had to say about "being on purpose." Leroy had noticed that. I then challenged him to use the interval between visits to discover his purpose. When he came back in about two weeks, he looked significantly better, as though the depression was about fifty percent relieved. He said that he had discovered that his purpose in life was to warn the young men in jail about the futility of trying to find happiness and fulfillment through violence and drug dealing, and to show them a different way that would work. As a senior convicted drug dealer, he had instant credibility with them, a distinct asset for a formidable challenge.

When I saw him again two or three weeks later, the depression was almost gone. He told me that the flashbacks to the horrors of combat in Vietnam were diminishing. He said that he had begun to talk with other prisoners about the concepts in *Real Magic*, including purpose in life and the happiness and fulfillment that comes as a result of "being on purpose." He had begun a discussion group in the cellblock. At first, he had an audience of one or two young men, and sometimes none at all. Soon, several were regularly listening to him. By that time, he knew something new and powerfully beneficial was going on in his life.

At the next visit, he was free of depression. He radiated a sense of excitement and a powerful awareness that something miraculous was happening. I had never seen anything remotely like this in him before. He was glowing with happiness. It was hard to believe that the broken hulk of a human being who had first been brought to the mental health center was the same person as this vibrant, self confident, happy man. Leroy sat and spoke with animation and joy about his adventures in mission fulfillment. He told me that the discussion group had grown from zero to three to standing room only. Practically everybody in the cellblock was attending.

The atmosphere on the cellblock was changing. Previously, the tension had been so high that Leroy never knew when violence would erupt. He did know that several of the prisoners had managed to manufacture knives, which they carried in case they were attacked, or decided they wanted to assault someone. The cellblock had been like a cage of starving animals, always on the verge of attacking one another. Over a period of weeks, this changed so much that the prisoners were offering to help one another, inviting another person to step ahead in the chow line and expressing care and concern for one another.

The new spirit of civility was important enough to them that when a surly new prisoner was brought in, the others would give him an opportunity to change his attitude. When he spoke or acted with violence or hatred, they would look at him in a way that was likely to make him ashamed. Peer pressure was sufficiently intense that most of the newcomers changed their attitudes and behavior. When one failed to do so, the other prisoners would say to a guard, "Get this dude out of here! He's messing up our cell block." The new prisoner would be removed. After telling me about this, Leroy looked at me with a twinkle in his eye and said, "Doc, *Real Magic* is loose in Dougherty County jail!"

I had to take Leroy's word for that, but I could see that *Real Magic* was loose in Leroy's life. I had never before seen such a magical change in a person in so short a time.

Leroy's metamorphosis was reminiscent of Viktor Frankl's account of how the power of purpose kept him alive in Nazi concentration camps. Frankl's book, *Man's Search for Meaning*, is the most gripping account we know of the importance of knowing and fulfilling mission.

DISCOVERING YOUR LIFE PURPOSE

In the previous chapter, we considered how to discover your Higher Self. Once you have met your Higher Self, however briefly, it becomes easier to answer the second big question: Why am I here? Even if you have never caught a glimpse of your Higher Self, in the gaps between your thoughts or anywhere else, you can still discover your purpose, but it will be more difficult and it may take longer. In that case, when you are beginning to discover your purpose and to take action to fulfill it, you become more likely to meet your Higher Self. It can work either way, but the easier way is to make at least some brief acquaintance with Higher Self first.

It may be that your most important purpose for being in this existence is to discover your Higher Self, since doing so marks the end of the kind of ignorance that is particularly deadly to the 100 year healthspan and to your quality of life every day. Therefore, you may want to identify as part of your mission in this life the discovery of your Higher Self. If that doesn't interest you, consider Dyer's assertion that one's basic purpose in life is to love unconditionally and serve other people.

Unconditionally loving means to serve without expectation of anything in return. The very idea of doing this sends ego into a frenzy of rage and outrage, yet doing it anyway is an amazingly liberating experience that saves incredible amounts of energy, trouble, and stress. Assuming the second jury was correct, consider the amount of energy, trouble, and stress that would have been avoided had O.J. Simpson unconditionally loved and served Nicole Brown Simpson, without expectation of anything in return. If this strikes you as a strange concept, take a few minutes to think about it. Try to imagine how your life would be different if this were your way of relating to others. Do you think that if you had no expectations of any other person there might be less disappointment and more fulfillment in your life?

If you decide to accept Dyer's position, the next question becomes "How do I serve others?" Chopra asserts, in the chapter on Dharma in *The Seven Spiritual Laws of Success*, that each person has some talent or group of talents that enables him or her to do something better than anyone else in the world can do it, or to exercise those talents in a particular way. For each particular expression of talent, there is a need somewhere by someone—and usually in many places by many people. Bringing the talent to the people who need it is an important part of mission fulfillment. Chopra recommends using the following steps to accomplish this:

Make a list of your unique talents and of things you love to do in the process of fulfilling those talents. If you cannot immediately think what those talents are, the realization will probably come to you during your times of quiet alertness, or shortly afterward. Whenever the realization comes, make the list. Then, each day ask yourself, "How can I help; how can I serve each person that I meet today?" As you do this, your energy will shift, you will feel lighter, freer, and be astonished at the opportunities that will unexpectedly open up for you to fulfill your mission.

With each action you take to fulfill mission, some happiness and additional energy will flow into your life. Part of this happiness is that you will feel the pressure of time lift from you. You will experience timeless awareness, which is a delicious experience of freedom and bliss. Another part of the happiness that you experience is the knowledge that you are providing others with something that they need, and doing it in a way that only you can provide. As you do this, exactly what you need for your own fulfillment and increased happiness will flow to you. It may not be what you expect; but if you set aside your expectations, or better yet, have no expectations in the first place, you will accept what comes and it will bless your life beyond anything you could expect. It may not happen immediately, and you may not understand it at the time, but it will happen and you will eventually understand and be glad and grateful.

SPECIFIC TECHNOLOGIES FOR THE DISCOVERY OF PURPOSE

You can use some specific technologies for discovery of purpose. Although they are different and one will suit you better than the others, they all have one thing in common: the experience of quiet alertness. Therefore, these technologies are different ways of focusing attention to achieve the experience of quiet alertness. One way is contemplation of nature.

When I was in my teens and experiencing a miserable amount of anger and paranoia, I would take long walks through a wilderness of sand ridges and scrub oak adjacent to the Alapaha River, where my parents owned a cabin. On long, hot, south Georgia afternoons, I walked for hours along old logging roads through this wilderness. As the hours and the miles passed, my mind gradually became quiet and I became one with the sand, the trees, the shimmering heat, the warm summer afternoon breeze, the rhythmic motion of walking, and the soft swish of sand underfoot. All of the anger, paranoia, and disturbance were left behind. Instead, there was the wonderful, refreshing blessing of quiet alertness. I craved these times as a man perishing of thirst craves a long drink of pure, cool water. I returned to the sand ridges whenever I could for the only relief I could find from the mental suffering of my daily life.

Years later, in the early seventies I was putting my life back together after wrecking it with destructive things I had done during a decade of abusing alcohol. I then found that I could experience the same timeless awareness and restful alertness by paddling a canoe in the river near the cabin before daybreak. Whenever I could arrange to spend the night at the cabin, I would get up while the stars were still bright, push the canoe out into the river and slowly paddle in the leisurely current as the stars paled, the sky turned gray, and dawn appeared. During the hour or so that I spent in this way, there was always the same experience of quiet alertness that blessed my life just as it had done on those long walks on the sand ridges years before. On the river, my attention was focused on the magic and splendor of daybreak in a wild and natural place.

One morning, after I had paddled down the river for a half-mile or so, I turned the canoe and paddled back upstream against the gentle current. The stars had faded; the sky had changed from black to gray to blue. The mellow fragrance of the river swamp at dawn was in the air. Then the first rays of the morning sun touched the tops of the tall pines and cypress on the west bank of the river. The hush of the sunrise was on the river and the surrounding woods. My attention was completely absorbed in the beauty and enchantment of the early morning. No thought stirred in my mind. Everything disappeared except the breathtaking perfection of nature, the sunrise and the rhythm of the paddle pushing against the water on the left side of the canoe. At one particular moment, as the paddle came out of the water at the end of a stroke, I heard the musical sounds of water drops from the paddle blade striking the surface of the lake. In that moment, I suddenly understood how I was to fulfill the purpose of my life. It was to teach people what they needed to know in order to fulfill their potential as human beings. That would set us free from the problem of suffering.

Before that time, I had some vague understanding that the way to fulfill my purpose was something like that, but with the crystal clarity that came in that particular moment, my whole value system suddenly reoriented itself, becoming focused and clear. Feeling stunned by the power and the clarity of the experience, I paddled slowly up the river while my understanding of my life realigned itself. After a few minutes, when most of my feeling of disorientation and the gooseflesh had passed, I turned the canoe and paddled back to the cabin. From that moment onward, my life had a focus and a direction that had never been there before. The process of repairing the damage that I had done to my family, my practice, and myself accelerated. I was able to move on to do the things necessary to fulfill the purpose that had become as clear as that sunrise.

Absorption in natural beauty is a way that has been used by many to answer the question, "Why am I here?" The vision quest was a rite of passage from childhood to adulthood for people of many Native American tribes. The young person would go alone into the wilderness for several days to fast and meditate until the realization of identity and purpose came. Once perceived, it became the focus around which that individual organized his life. If you feel an affinity for Native American culture, you may want to consider a vision quest. It can be helpful to have a Native American shaman instruct and guide you in the process. If you can not find a shaman, you can get good guidance from your intellect and intuition, particularly when they are sharpened and brought into balance by the regular experience of quiet alertness. A few days alone in the wilderness may bring an understanding of purpose that it would otherwise take years or lifetimes to gain.

For those who prefer not to make such an extensive commitment of time and energy, but still want to clearly know their purpose, there are several other options. Here is one that we have used in Healthspan Workshops.

1. Do this protocol in a group if possible. The group generates energy that enables everyone to access the necessary knowledge more easily. It is also fun, once you have made some discoveries, to discuss them with others who are engaged in the same process. You probably know some people who want to

know their own answers to this big question and who would be interested in spending an evening or half a day searching for it in a group. If you cannot find a group or do not want to organize one, you can still search productively alone.

2. Find the quietest, most pleasant place possible. If you can find one that helps you feel quiet and alert at the same time, that is very favorable. Mountain tops, seashore and groves of big, old trees have that effect, but you can probably also find enclosed places that will be settling, serene, and conducive to quiet alertness and discovery of purpose.

3. Once you find a suitable place, sit in a comfortable chair with your spine erect, close your eyes, and breathe normally through your nose. On each exhalation, repeat a mantra or focus phrase silently to yourself. If you already have a mantra, use it. If not, use the phrase "My purpose" or "So hum". Think the first word on inhalation and the second on exhalation. Continue this until your thoughts begin to slow, the gaps between them get wider, and you find yourself feeling calmer and lighter. You are now probably in the "alpha state," which is conducive to left brain/right brain balance that helps you integrate intellect and intuition to discover purpose.

4. While still repeating your mantra, with your eyes closed, visualize a blank screen. You can make it white or any color you wish. Notice what appears on the screen, what thoughts go through your mind, and what feelings you experience. Just notice these things; do not dwell on anything you see, think, or feel. Let the scenes, thoughts, and feelings come and go like clouds floating across a summer sky. Do this as though you were watching a movie. You are not controlling what happens on the screen; you are just watching it.

5. After 15 or 20 minutes, stop this visualization and observation process. Immediately write down what you saw,

thought, and felt. Write quickly, without thinking about what you are writing. Once you have finished writing, look over what you have written. What does it tell you about your purpose? Write down what you have discovered.

6. If the answer to the question "What does this tell you about your purpose?" is "Nothing", do not be dismayed. If you were going to chop down a large oak tree, the tree probably would not fall the first time you swung the axe. Discovery of purpose is usually a large oak tree indeed, so you should be prepared to do this procedure more than once. Remember that it works better and faster if you can do it in a group, or in a power place such as a seashore, mountain peak, old-growth forest, energy vortex, or any other place where you feel unusually strong, creative energy. If none of these places is available to you, you can still get an excellent result if you persist in doing this process as often as possible at home. Setting aside half a day in which you repeat the above procedure three or four times can be very productive, with more insight coming to you with each repetition.

THE BIGGEST BANG FOR THE BUCK

Part of the mission of Healthspan Center is to bring the most useful knowledge and cost-effective interventions for the attainment of your natural birthright. We not only want you to discover your purpose; we want you to do it as quickly, easily, and economically as possible. From the experiences that I have described, as well as from the daily practice of meditation, I have learned something important about cost-effectiveness. Before I began to meditate, the only way I knew to experience quiet alertness was to go to the wilderness or to the river. Since I managed to do that only once or twice a month, there were some long dry spells between visits. I often thought of the lines in the Rubaiyat, "A momentary halt, a momentary taste of being from the well amidst the waste..." Those momentary tastes of being with long dry spells between were no more satisfactory than eating once or twice a month. One of the great joys and delights of learning to meditate was gaining the ability to experience every day the quiet alertness that I previously had been able to have only occasionally.

Having a procedure for discovering purpose that you can use practically anywhere has the same advantage. It might take you a long time to go on enough vision quests or journeys to mountaintops, seashores, or old growth forests to discover your purpose. Once you have these protocols, however, you can work on it every day and probably discover your answer far sooner.

If this protocol does not feel appealing to you, here are two other good ones. Dyer, in *Real Magic,* describes one. The pages in the paperback edition are 9 through 14. Intuitive people, who are accustomed to using right brain processes, generally like Dr. Dyer's protocol and the Healthspan protocol.

Left brain people, who want a more intellectual, analytical experience, may prefer a method of Dr. Stephen Covey. In *The Seven Habits of Highly Effective People,* Covey gives directions for going through a series of intellectual exercises that enable you to view your purpose in life, or mission, as he calls it, from several perspectives. Once you have done this, he gives instructions on writing your personal mission statement. You can even let your computer help you, if you run Microsoft Office 97, Professional Edition. One of the programs in the Office suite is Schedule +. Call up "Stephen Covey." You will find a program that will ask a series of questions. After you enter your answers, the computer will show you a draft of your personal mission statement. You can then revise it until it says exactly what you want it to.

Once you have your mission statement, it becomes your personal constitution by which you govern your life in much the same way the United States is supposed to be governed by the US Constitution. Whatever procedure you use, persist until you know your answer! This will spare you the chagrin of, as Covey says, spending decades and the strength and resources of your life climbing the ladder of success only to discover, upon arriving at the top, that it was leaning against the wrong wall.

Actually, you do not have to wait very long to discover your purpose. According to tradition, the Buddha once said, "Your work is to discover your work, and then with all your heart to give yourself to it." If this makes sense to you, you will never, from this moment forward, be without knowing your purpose in life. You will either be in the process of discovering your purpose, which is your current provisional purpose, or you will have discovered it. How quickly you discover your purpose will depend largely on how intensely you search. For fastest results, search with the same intensity that you would use when extinguishing a fire in your hair.

Once you have discovered your purpose, you will naturally want to fulfill it as efficiently and completely as possible. After all, doing so is the only reliable source of happiness in your life and one of the most powerful things for attaining your 100-year healthspan.

When I ask my patients about their purpose in life, some will say, "My purpose is to be happy." I usually tell them, "If your purpose is to be happy, you can't get there from here. Happiness doesn't come from trying to be happy. You may have some transient feelings of happiness but they are dependent on what another person does or the circumstances of your life. Depending on anyone but yourself for your happiness puts you in a very insecure, weak position. Happiness comes from being in the process of fulfilling your purpose. Once you know what your purpose in life is and begin to act to fulfill it, life will bring you opportunities every day to do so. Doors will unexpectedly open in what appeared to be blank walls. Once you are fulfilling purpose, 'Happiness will follow you as your shadow, unshakable,' as the Dhamma Pada says."

Not only is the fulfillment of purpose the only reliable source of happiness, but dying without fulfilling purpose is probably the ultimate horror. Ultimately, the choice of discovering and fulfilling purpose or not comes down to the choice between happiness and horror. We prefer happiness, and that is our wish for you.

THE PROOF OF THE PURPOSE PUDDING

"The proof of the pudding is in the eating," says an old proverb. The proof of the purpose pudding is in the living. If you think you know your life purpose, but you are not sure, try this test. Ask yourself, "Does doing the things I spend most of my time and energy on every day bring happiness into my life every day?" If the answer is, "Yes," or even, "Usually," the probability is high that you are "on purpose." Please notice that the question is *not*, "Is my life free of stress, challenge, pain, and struggle?" Any purpose worthy of you will probably bring all these experiences at times. The crucial question is whether, in spite of the stress, challenge, pain, and struggle, the happiness keeps on coming also. If you have not yet experienced this combination of painful struggle and happiness, you have an interesting and enlightening experience in store. We hope that you will have the experience soon.

Regularly experiencing happiness while in the process of doing things that also cause discomfort is a reliable reassurance that you really are "on purpose." This reassurance is not the only value of this experience of concurrent happiness and discomfort; it also gives you surprising strength and stress tolerance. The reliable, predictable daily input of happiness empowers you to continue to function effectively under stress that would otherwise overwhelm you. Longfellow wrote about "... that fierce joy that warriors feel / in foemen worthy of their steel." A warrior filled with fierce joy is more likely to come home *with* his shield than *on* it.

FULFILLING YOUR MISSION

Once you know, even partially, what your mission is, you will want to begin to fulfill it as effectively as possible. Here are five things that will enable you to do so.

1. Develop your personal mission statement, using the method of Covey in *The Seven Habits of Highly Effective People*, pages 96 through 144. Alternatively, use the program in Schedule + of Microsoft Office 97, Professional Edition. As mentioned earlier, your mission statement then becomes your constitution, or compass, that helps you stay on course for the fulfillment of purpose in spite of the stresses, distractions and vicissitudes of daily life. One of the most important things about the mission statement is that it helps you maintain balance among the various roles that you must play in order to fulfill your mission. In addition to being useful, you may find the process fascinating and fun.

2. After developing your mission statement, connect with an inexhaustible source of energy and intelligence for unlimited fulfillment. You can do this by using the technology of James Redfield, which he presents in *The Celestine Prophecy, The Tenth Insight,* and the experiential guides to those books. In 1997, *The Celestine Prophecy* had, for the past two years, been the largest selling book in the world. CBS is in the process of making it into a four-hour television special. In these books, Redfield presents the systematic process for connecting with the intelligence and energy that runs the universe. I think of it as a way of establishing a solid connection with the Field of Pure Consciousness.

Once you have this connection, fulfillment of purpose increases beyond what would ever be possible otherwise. The process of fulfillment will be strongly supported by fortunate occurrences that Redfield calls synchronicities. I will presently give some examples of these synchronicities, but first, the remainder of the recommendations.

3. Plan each week, using the Planner and protocol developed by Covey. Information about this Planner and its protocol, as well as the Planner itself, is available from Franklin Covey. See Resources for phone and website. You can multiply your effectiveness many times by spending thirty minutes at the beginning of the week reviewing your mission statement and the roles that you must fill in accomplishing your mission. Then, you can more skillfully decide and plan how you will use the available time and energy during the week for most efficient mission fulfillment. This process also helps to maintain balance in your life, since you are much less likely to get so preoccupied with fulfilling one role that you neglect others that are equally important.

4. In addition to planning your week at the beginning of each week, consider planning your month on the day of each new moon. Gordon-Michael Scallion, a prominent futurist, believes that this is a particularly favorable time to make plans for the month. I have followed his recommendation and agree that it is helpful.

5. Finally, set aside the last eight hours of December 31st, the last day of the year, to review your adventures in being on purpose in the past year and set your goals for the coming year. We call this event a New Year's Eve Quest. It is best done with family and close friends. It has been a tradition in our family every New Year's Eve since 1973.

A SCINTILLATING SEQUENCE OF CELESTINE SYNCHRONICITIES

We think of the process through which we came to Rabun County as a scintillating sequence of synchronicities. The sequence actually has no beginning and no end, but we will describe briefly thirty-two years of it, beginning with the day, previously mentioned, when I bought a copy of *Zen Buddhism*, in the Miami Airport. As you already know, Jack III spoke the words in 1975 that opened the book for me. The following year, Roshi Kapleau accepted me as his student. I was fully committed to Zen practice, so when the Roshi decided to build a Zen Center in the mountains west of Denver, I closed my practice, put the office and the house on the market, and was preparing to move to Denver to participate in that project.

Then, interest rates reached 20% and the Roshi decided that was not the time to borrow millions of dollars to build the Zen Center. Since I had closed my practice and had little income, I went to work as the medical director of the local mental health center.

In 1982, we discovered Andy had cancer. In the following two years his medical bills probably approached $100,000. The family had excellent health insurance through my employment. Never before or since have we had insurance that covered virtually all medical expenses. Never before or since has there been such a great need for such coverage.

In 1990, Roshi Kapleau sent me a copy of *Quantum Healing* by Chopra. This led me to ayurvedic physician's training in 1991 and to doing ayurvedic consultations at the TM Center in Atlanta, starting in 1992. Although I recognized that ayurveda was the ideal framework for the practice of holistic medicine, the culture of Southwest Georgia was not very receptive to that system. In fact, I often felt like a rabbi reciting psalms in a mosque. This made the Atlanta consultations very welcome.

In 1993, I received a call from an orthodontist in Atlanta who was establishing a holistic health center. One of my Atlanta patients had told him about my work. He invited me to serve as medical director of the new center, to make sure it developed a truly holistic program. I was delighted to begin to work part-time in that facility.

While serving there, I met an orthopedic surgeon who was a consultant to the Center. He invited us to his office in the foothills of the northeast Georgia mountains to see patients once a month. We were delighted to do this, too. He and his wife opened their home to us and we became close friends.

In July 1994, the Great Flood destroyed the Wellness Center in Albany where I was practicing holistic medicine part time, while continuing to see patients at the mental health center. After that disaster, the North Georgia practices were even more valuable and attractive. During one of our visits, the orthopedic surgeon suggested that I talk with the psychiatrist who was the medical director of a psychiatric hospital nearby. By then, we knew that it was time to move to the north Georgia mountains, so I followed my friend's suggestion. I learned that the medical director was interested in holistic medicine and wanted to discuss the possibility of my doing some inservice training for the hospital staff. I arrived for that discussion one day in January 1995. On the way to a meeting with some other members of the hospital staff, the medical director said that he had just resigned his position and the hospital was in urgent need of another psychiatrist. Within two months, we had moved to Rabun County, where I worked at the psychiatric hospital, began a part time private practice, and started writing this book. In the spring of 1996, I had fulfilled my agreement to work at that hospital for a year. They had found a full time psychiatrist and it was time for me to devote my energies to my growing holistic medical practice and the book.

Since we have been in Rabun County, we have met several people who have been of great help in our mission fulfillment. Our friendship with the orthopedic surgeon and his wife has grown deeper and more inspiring. We met Martin Wuttke, one of the pioneers in the development of neurofeedback technologies for the expansion of consciousness. He and I have consulted on a number of patients who were so sick that it is doubtful that either or us alone could have been of much help. With the combination of holistic medicine and neurofeedback, a remarkably large number of these patients have made breathtaking recoveries.

We met a registered nurse who is a master of therapeutic touch. We have had consultations about many difficult patients who have gone on to make more progress than would have been likely without the combined effort. We also met an astrologer who, from his charts, told me the procedures that I should follow to facilitate the writing of the book. I cannot imagine the project's developing as well as it has without this guidance.

As we look back over the thirty-two years since 1965, we know that these key events are synchronicities and not mere coincidences. We know that there is an Intelligence that has guided this whole process, is guiding it today and will guide it for as long as it needs to continue, provided we follow faithfully the guidance that comes to us and remain dedicated to the fulfillment of purpose. There is nothing unique about this guidance process. It is a principal theme of *The Celestine Prophecy* and *The Tenth Insight*. We have talked with many people who have had similar experiences. In fact, we have not talked with anyone who is seriously dedicated to fulfilling mission who does not receive this kind of guidance and synchronistic assistance. The guidance may not come and the doors may not open as soon as we think they should and wish they would, but it comes and they open when the time is right. Later, we see that. Life has to be lived forward and understood backwards. As a wise child once remarked while riding a train in a rearward facing seat, "This is like life: I can see where I've been, but not where I'm going."

If you are not already experiencing this, you will, when you dedicate yourself to answering your Big Questions and living out the answers in the details of your daily life. The more passionately you commit yourself to the fulfillment of mission, the more frequently these synchronicities occur.

Soon after I went into psychiatric practice, a new patient remarked, "Doc, I am going to be well—or bust hell wide open." That spirit brings on the surprising synchronicities and stunning success in mission fulfillment. Thoreau wrote, "If a man advances confidently in the direction of his dreams and endeavors to live the life that he has imagined, he will meet with success unexpected in common hours." Goethe said, "Whatever you can do, or dream you can, begin it. Boldness has genius, power and magic in it." If you follow their advice, you will find that they spoke truth. We have tried it for over twenty years; it has not failed yet. It never will.

Without this sequence of synchronicities that supported our move from the southwest Georgia flatlands to the northeast Georgia mountains, we would not have made the move. We would have stayed stuck in southwest Georgia, where mission fulfillment would have been mediocre, at best. The determination to fulfill purpose at all costs plays well over time.

The Buddhist definition for the middle way does not mean compromise; it means higher, like the apex of a triangle. In searching for a higher way, two people must find a solution that is better than what either person presently has in mind.
—The Covey Seven Habits Organizer

Chapter 10

WHO ARE ALL THESE OTHERS?

"It is your fault that Andy died," my father told Jack during his visit at the nursing home only days after the memorial service. "God is punishing you for being a member of a cult."

We had made no secret of the fact that most of the family had learned to do Zen meditation and were doing it. Dad always had "the truth". Anyone who did not subscribe to his beliefs was therefore wrong, and sinning — and he had the scripture to prove it.

Four years previously, when it became evident that Dad could no longer live in his home in Kentucky because of the tension between him and his wife's family, Jack lovingly opened our home and his heart to Dad when none of the my siblings and their spouses either could or would take him in. What impressed me most about the way that Jack reacted to this devastating accusation that Dad had made was that it did not change in any way his relationship with Dad. Jack continued visiting him regularly in the nursing home, engaging him in stimulating conversation, and letting Dad know that he loved and cared for him. In so far as I could tell, Jack handled the situation as if it had never happened; he still loved my Dad unconditionally and was able to communicate that by word and deed when he visited him.

Dad died a very slow death — much like a mushroom's drying out and being gradually blown away in the wind — so it was impossible to tell just when the moment of death might come. He was 93 years old and apparently had no diagnosable illness. On a

December Sunday morning while I was at church playing for the Christmas program, Jack visited Dad. As he left, he put his hand on Dad's hand and said, "Travel freely, undisturbed." Dad died late that afternoon. Jack took the same loving, compassionate care of my Dad that he had taken of his own father.

The Christian scriptures admonish us to love our neighbors as we love ourselves. What does this mean? Perhaps it means that we can love others only to the extent that we love ourselves. For this reason, it is exceedingly important to learn first to love and respect ourselves — just as we are — imperfect with freckles, knock- knees, a hot temper, whatever. This does not mean that we stop trying to improve ourselves. It does mean that we learn to respect ourselves enough to take care of our basic human needs and that we *behave* in such a way that respecting ourselves becomes a way of life. When I respect myself, I respect you. When I love myself, it is easier for me to love you. Review the chapter "Who am I?" for suggestions on how to establish the foundation of all relationships — love and respect for self.

MANAGING NEGATIVE EMOTIONS

Unfortunately, much energy is wasted in relationships by harboring ill feelings, resentment, and anger. Who is getting hurt when feelings of anger and resentful are carefully nurtured? The one holding the grudge! The other person may not even be aware of what she has done that has been displeasing. There is a Zen saying that we are not punished *for* our anger; we are punished *by* it. An interesting thing that I learned during my year of clinical training in TA is that when my anger surfaces, it is nearly always triggered by my own not OK feelings about myself, my feelings of inferiority.

Eric Berne, M.D. wrote many interesting books; one of the most popular was *Games People Play*. Unfortunately some people in close relationships play a psychological game that Berne called, "Now I Have Got You, You Son of a Bitch!" How does one play this game?

A beautiful woman came in for counseling because her husband of 20 years had asked her for a divorce. In trying to discover why he wanted to leave—she thought the marriage was good—she was willing to listen to his dissatisfaction with the relationship. He told her that, starting very early in the marriage, she had told him how to run his business and what he should do about every situation. Instead of kindly telling her that he would like for her to listen to his problems without giving him any advice, he very carefully hid the anger in his heart, something like putting a drop of water into a bucket.

After 20 years of feeling that she had discounted his ability to solve problems every time she gave him advice, his emotional "bucket" ran over. She assured him that she was sorry and that she could change. "It is too late," he replied; "I have already found someone else." This was a particularly heartbreaking divorce because two teenage children were involved. However, this divorce did not need to happen! Had the husband known how to take care of his resentments as they occurred, the wife would have probably been motivated to change her behavior. As it was, she had no idea that a wound was festering in his heart.

In most of the divorce cases in which I have been involved, one person has taken emotional abuse or has been dissatisfied with the relationship for years without telling the other about the discomfort. Most of us do not have the skill to sit down with the other partner during a period of calm and say what needs changing in the relationship. Instead, we keep the feelings bottled up until we reach the boiling point. At that point, our pain comes out as poison instead of a plea for change. Too often, the dissatisfied one becomes involved in another relationship before the other partner has much awareness that something is wrong.

For those of us who have problems keeping our cool while discussing deeply emotional issues, I recommend putting the grievances on paper to be given to the significant other. I also recommend that the "hurting" one put in as many positives as she can. Sandwiching the grievances between two sets of things one appreciates about the other person helps to put him or her in a more cooperative frame of mind.

Does this mean that we go around spouting off all negative feelings every time they occur? Of course not! Many times the negative feelings we have are inappropriate. I remember all too clearly the day that Andy brought home a bad report card. My first impulse was to vent my anger and disappointment at Andy for not spending more time on his studies and less time with his friends. I realized that this feeling of anger towards Andy was inappropriate. Several years before this incident, I had decided that, when my guts were tied in knots, it was time to excuse myself and go for a walk if it was daytime. If it was after dark, it was time to go to my room to meditate and get myself under control before confronting the child. What I discovered that afternoon while I was walking was that I had a recording in my head that said, "If you are a good mother, your children will make good grades." According to that recording, I was a failure as a mother — and the anger was really towards myself, not Andy. Fortunately, I realized that that recording was inappropriate and decided to get rid of it.

First, before expressing angry feelings to someone about your dissatisfaction with him, get your mind calm and clear. See whether this anger is appropriate. If it is appropriate, and sometimes it is, the confrontation still needs to be done with kindness. It also needs to be done one on one, no one else present. The expectation needs to be clearly spelled out. Sometimes it is appropriate to also spell out what the consequences will be if the behavior does not change. For instance, it was appropriate for me to tell Andy that his television time or play time after school would be shortened until he brought his grades up, but it would not have been appropriate to have taken out my anger on him.

FORGIVENESS

We all have someone in our lives that we need to forgive — a parent, a friend, a child, a neighbor. Unfortunately, forgiveness is a skill that few people possess. What does it mean to forgive? Even as children we were taught that the Christian way is to forgive and forget. What happens when we try to "forget" something? We cannot get the memory of that incident out of the mind! When a person says that she has forgiven someone but still brings up the situation, it is probable that forgiveness has not taken place. Instead of trying to forget a painful situation, do what needs to be done to defuse the negative feelings towards the other person. Here are some suggestions that we have found useful:

1. Go back and review the situation that needs to be forgiven. What part did I play in this situation? What could I have done differently that would have made the outcome of this situation better? Do I need first to forgive myself for not handling this situation skillfully? Was there something that I needed to have said or done that was left out?

2. Every time that the painful memory emerges, send love to the other person.

3. If the person who has wronged you lives nearby, do something thoughtful for that person; for example, making them some muffins, taking them a fruit basket, or a load of firewood.

4. Do visual imagery. Sit in a comfortable chair. Close your eyes and take several deep breaths. When the body is relaxed and the mind is clear, visualize something great happening to the other person. Would this person like more material goods? Visualize an abundance of material goods coming their way. Do they need a physical healing? Visualize your love going into their body to help with the healing.

5. Remind yourself that relationships are made up of human beings who are imperfect. Accept the imperfections of others while also accepting our own.

6. If it is appropriate, apologize to the other person for the part that you played in the painful situation.

7. Do not even attempt to forget the painful situation. After you have forgiven the person and yourself for the problem, mentally make a file in your head with the year and the date on it. File the incident away, remembering that it is a forgiven incident.

PROBLEM SOLVING

There is another important way to keep tension down in relationships. Learning to be a good listener is a skill all of us need and few possess. Asking the "right" questions is also important. Someone you love has brought a problem to you. Are they asking you to solve the problem? Probably not! They may just need someone to listen to them, to mirror back to them what they are struggling with. The sequence that I have found useful in helping people with problems is:

1. First, define the problem. Oftentimes this is the hardest part of the conversation. Once you have repeated to the other person what you think the problem is, he may decide that what he has communicated is not really the problem at all. Your listening is helping him to define the problem. Once, when Jack was interviewing a couple, the husband insisted that his wife was having an affair because she had started wearing earrings. When Jack repeated to him what he had just said, the husband realized how absurd his accusation was.

2. Who owns the problem? Make sure that you are not trying to solve a problem that is not your problem. For example a woman who deeply wants to have only love, peace and

harmony in her family sometimes brings to me problems that her daughter is having with her husband. This woman does not seem to realize that the tension between her daughter and her husband belongs to *them* and is not a problem that she can solve. She can listen to them attentively and affirm her love and affection for them, but she cannot solve their problems. She has the option of course, of worrying herself sick about the problem she can not solve!

3. What options does the person see as solutions to the problem? After you have listened to the options, share with him any others that you may see. In working with teenagers, always remember that one option they may see is suicide. If the problem is a severe one, I often ask for a no-suicide contract with the other person. I ask them to make a contract with me that they will not die of natural or unnatural causes without discussing it with me first. Only one client has refused to make that contract — and in the years when I was in the counseling practice, I had to return to the office many times on weekends and after hours to listen to what the other person needed to say before she committed suicide. It worked. Not once did a client see the situation as hopeless and kill herself.

4. What do you see as the consequences of your taking option X, Y, or Z?

5. Which options will work best? It helps to keep in mind that *there are some problems to which there are no perfect solutions*. We need to take the option that our hearts tell us would affect the other people involved and ourselves in the best or least harmful way.

Please note that, if you follow some line of questioning similar to what we have outlined, you do not assume the responsibility of solving that person's problem. As Jack has often told me, "The supply of advice far exceeds the demand!" Learn to listen so attentively that the person who has brought to you a problem sees the problems and options for resolving the problem. This way of working on problems is a particularly great asset when the children are teenagers. When we really learn to listen to them without giving advice, they are much more likely to listen to us.

As I learned to listen to our children while they were adolescents without giving them advice or mentioning options until they had finished their position, I sometimes changed my position on the problem. This also happens in the business world.

The importance of our relationships with others was beautifully expressed in the first movie, "Oh, God!" The character played by John Denver reminded God of all the heartaches, disappointments and messes we were making of our lives here on earth and asked God why he did not come to dwell among us again in physical form. God replied, "I have given you each other!"

THREE REQUIREMENTS

It helps to keep in mind these three requirements to having healthy, fulfilling, creative relationships:

1. The *will* to make the relationship work. If there is not a commitment to the relationship, when problems arise — and they will—it is easier to sever the relationship than it is to try to work out the problems. When the bride walks down the aisle thinking that, if this relationship does not work out the way she wants it to (or expects it to), then she will get a divorce, do not put any money on that relationship's becoming a marriage of mature love! A handsome thirty-something man was telling me about the stress he was having with his newfound love. He sighed and said, "Oh, well, if this relationship is meant to work, it will." Hogwash! The relationship probably will not work unless he is committed to working it out and to learning the skills he needs to know in order to solve problems as they come. (The relationship crumbled.)

2. The *skills* to make the relationship a quality one—not just a commitment to staying together. A few of the skills needed are mentioned in this chapter, but space does not permit our going into the details we need to master to raise the level of loving acceptance. A subsequent book on relationships will cover the skills more completely.

3. *Time.* During courtship we willingly listen to the beloved all night if need be. After the vows are spoken, too few people take the prime time that is necessary to make a relationship a loving one. One reason that Jack and I are together—and enjoying a high level of love and respect and a low level of tension—is that, from the very first when we were married in 1954, we have taken at least two hours every week to do fun things together or just talk. This was particularly important when the children were young. Then, Jack was working Wednesdays and Saturdays until noon and we could usually get someone to keep the children on Wednesday for us to have a "date".

When the children were young, Jack instigated a ritual of spending at least two hours one Friday night a month with each child—alone. The child got to choose what he/she would do during that time. Our younger son always wanted to ride motorcycles, so Jack bought a used motorcycle and rode with him on Sunday afternoons instead of Friday night. Our daughter always wanted to go shopping. Jack willingly took her to the lingerie department and helped her shop. Jack's willingness to spend some of his precious time, while he was maintaining a very busy psychiatric practice, conveyed to each child the important place each held in his life. These visits also opened communication with the child on such a deep level that they always knew that they could discuss any issue with their Dad. His relationship with our daughter also set the stage for the kind of man she looked for when she decided in her late 20's that it was time to look for a soul mate. Since her Dad and brothers had always treated her with love and respect (except for the time that she and our older son were both going through puberty. At that point, I thought they might kill each other!), it was very difficult for her to find a male in her generation that would treat her in the manner to which she had become accustomed.

All too often in our modern, stress-filled lives, we work hard developing a relationship until the vows are spoken. Then we breathe a sigh of relief that we have accomplished what we set out to do. Now we put our time and energies into developing the business, raising children or whatever else our lives bring to us. The marriage is now a done deal; it will take care of itself. But it does not. We would not even consider buying a business, then walking off to let it take care of itself; yet that is exactly what we do in our close relationships.

We first learn from our families of origin or from the people who raised us what to do in close relationships. The theory is, and I believe that it is valid, that any problem that our parents did not resolve in their relationships, we "inherit" to work out in our own relationships. I never saw my mother and father even discuss a problem. Whatever father wanted, father got. If we children disagreed with him, it was called "talking back" and he often punished us. Whatever Dad thought was "right" was never questioned, so it was very difficult for me to learn to confront problems instead of sweeping them under the carpet and then manifesting a physical symptom as my mother had done. It is true that families repeat their history in later generations. This is based at least partly on the lack of problem solving skills. Consequently, the same problems show up generation after generation.

Let us encourage you to work out the problems in your close relationships although you may have decided to leave the relationship. This is particularly helpful if there are children, even grown children, involved. If you do not learn what you need to learn about resolving the problem that you have in your present relationship, you will no doubt get the opportunity to work it out in a later relationship. In other words, the problem will probably come back to haunt you!

BOWEN'S FAMILY SYSTEMS THEORY

There came a time in our relationship when we needed professional help. Although it appeared to me that the marriage was not salvageable, there were three children who had not asked to be born. We believed that the children deserved an intact family—one able to nurture and support them financially and emotionally until they were at least 18 years old. We first consulted a local psychiatrist. He gave me a handful of Elavil and sent us on our way. On the second day on the Elavil, I had the insight that Jack was just as much the problem as I was, and he got no medication! So I flushed the remaining Elavil down the commode and decided to start attending all the psychiatric training sessions with Jack.

During these years that I was an empty vessel searching for ways to deal with my emotional problems, we attended training sessions by Virginia Satir and many other notables in the field of family and couple's therapy. It was not until we attended a symposium at Georgetown University on Family Systems Theory that we finally found the tools with which to make not just a good marriage, but a great one. (Dr. Murray Bowen later called his theory Bowen Family Systems Theory, when so many other family systems theories were being taught. Basically, his theory teaches how to deal with the "craziness" in the family without having to leave the family.) Space does not permit a complete overview of the system, but here are a few things that we were able to put to immediate use in our family.

Any time there is trouble or stress in adult relationships, each person needs to take the responsibility for his/her part. So many times, it appears that ONE person is the one to blame; the other is innocent. That is very seldom so. It is accurate to say that, anytime there is stress in an adult/adult relationship, the responsibility for the stress rests about 50% on each person. An example is a man in his late 50's. He is severely depressed at times. His wife is the functioning head of the family. The man "swallows" anger towards his wife but never confronts her. Yet, he is 50% responsible for the relationship — for causing the problem and for solving it. (Please note the use of the word "responsibility". It is usually counterproductive to assign "fault" in relationship problems.)

One of the first and most important things that I learned from Dr. Bowen was, "The way to control children is to control yourself!" (No hitting or lashing out in anger.) O.K., I thought. Dr. Bowen obviously does not know 13 year old Jack III who then had raging hormones to go along with his hot temper. The usual scenario between Jack III and me was for him to come to the kitchen while I was preparing dinner and angrily accuse me of "hiding" his hammer (he loved to build things with his hands). Usually he was screaming at me at this point, and I screamed back at him to get out of the kitchen; couldn't he see that I was busy?! Then the two of us were off and running on a screaming fight. Although I had no inkling that Dr. Bowen was right, I nonetheless realized that something had to be done; otherwise, I may have to do physical harm to J. III before he turned 14 and he was already larger than I was.

One day I sat the children down and told them that I was going to try getting myself calm before I dealt with problems I was having with them. If I needed to, I would leave the house and go walking until I calmed down, but I would be back and would deal with the problem when I could do it calmly. Over the next few months I developed good, strong leg muscles, but I did keep my word about not losing my cool. At first, J.III tried me out—and that was predictable. The next time he came into the kitchen screaming that I had misplaced his hammer, I calmly told him that I would be glad to help him look for the hammer once I was through mashing the potatoes. A miracle began to occur! J.III quit screaming at me! In fact, by the time he turned sixteen, his hot temper had totally abated. I have not seen him loose his cool from that point to this! Granted, both Jack and I were working hard at that point on getting control of self (NOT repressing feelings, but really getting control). Did Jack III learn to control himself just by watching us learn to control ourselves? It was an important key to bringing down the stress between our teenage children and us.

Now, when we hear parents complain about the problems of having teenagers in the house, we remember that the home does not have to be a war zone between parents and teenagers. Parents need to do their part in changing the relationship more in the direction of an adult/adult relationship. That means allowing the teenagers to make whatever decisions they can make while the parents are there to backstop them if they make an unskillful decision. Parents do not offer unsolicited advice. Bowen said that the ideal parent-child relationship was one in which the parent is there when the child needs him or her, and the rest of the time stays out of the child's way.

The parents also need to know that the children relate to the *relationship* between the parents and that the best thing that they can do for the children is to have a friendly relationship with each other, regardless of whether the relationship is called marriage, divorce, living together, whatever. All too often, parents try to get a child to "side" with them against the other parent, thereby creating an unhealthy triangle where a child has to carry some of the burden of the parents' immaturity.

In the years that we spent learning Bowen's Family Systems Theory, we learned that, in every marriage, one person gives up more of his/her self than the other person. In other words, one person becomes the "functioning self " while the other person becomes the "adapted self." The person who is the functioning self is usually the comfortable one. The one who has given up levels of self (sometimes also one's last name, one's geographical location or one's family) becomes the uncomfortable one and is much more subject to physical, emotional or social illnesses. Unfortunately, the uncomfortable one does not usually discuss the discomfort with the other. They put up with the discomfort until it becomes poison in the relationship, the perfect set-up for some form of physical or emotional illness, or an affair.

Dr. Bowen recommends that, instead of opting out of the relationship, each person work on developing a higher level of solid self in the relationship. This is most skillfully done by first doing what Dr. Bowen calls, "differentiating a self in one's family or origin." Why start there? Because it was in our family of origin that we learned to adapt, it was there that we developed a small level of solid self and usually a huge level of what Dr. Bowen calls "pseudo-self". Basically, what he recommends is learning to take an "I" position with one's parents, siblings, etc. by starting first at the outer edge of the family and learning to take an "I" position with aunts, uncles and cousins. As we learn to do that skillfully, it is then easier to take an "I" position with one's parents and siblings. At that point, it is then easier to take an "I" position with one's significant other. (An "I" position is taken calmly with no emotional overtones. It is easier for beginners if they begin every sentence with "I".)

This was a particularly difficult assignment for me. Mother had dropped dead from an apparent heart attack when I was 26 years old. My father was something of a tyrant. He was always right; no one disagreed with him unless she was willing to have the wrath of God called down upon her—a scary situation. The first time that I took an "I" position with Dad, I was sitting across from him at the breakfast table. Dad made some remark—one of his truths. I listened attentively to him, then carefully repeated to him what I had heard. Dad said that I had heard him right; that was "the truth." I then stated my position, kindly, a position that was different from his. Dad's chin dropped. He could not believe that one of his children had disagreed with him. With fire in his eyes he leaned across the table, pointed his finger at me, and said, "The devil has you right where he wants you!" Years earlier, I would have recoiled in horror to this statement. Now I accepted it without being frightened of what he might do to me.

There is power in a family system that can heal or destroy. The Bowen System teaches how to better turn the system around to be a system of love instead of one of destruction. For a systematic presentation of Bowen's work, see his book, *Family Therapy in Clinical Practice.*

THE HEALING POWER OF LOVE

As stated earlier, love is the most powerful healing energy that we know. This makes it vital to the attainment of healthy, happy, fulfilling relationships and the 100-year healthspan. Since we live in a spectacularly "suboptimal" environment, we get hurt frequently, which means we need a lot of healing. If you need a lot of healing, it makes sense to find the most effective healing energy possible. That is love. Relationships offer the most important opportunities for the manifestation of love. To make the most of that opportunity, it is important to answer the third big question, "Who are all these other people in my life and what is the true nature of my relationship to them?" If you first understand the nature of the relationship, it becomes much easier to learn who the people are. With that accomplished, the way is open for the cultivation and manifestation of love in your relationships.

Some configurations of relationships are more favorable for the manifestation of love than others. Marriage is one of the more important of these. Marriage has some disadvantages, but it also has great advantages for the attainment of the 100-year healthspan. In fact, married people live longer than singles.

One of the advantages of marriage is that it is a sure cure for a prevalent form of temporary insanity called "being in love." Being in love is a type of temporary insanity characterized by the delusion that your beloved is going to make you happy. Although this can be a severe form of derangement, and can lead to extraordinarily bizarre behavior, it is temporary because it is readily cured by marriage. Sometimes living together will cure it, but marriage is the sure cure. Once the temporary insanity is cured, the way is cleared for the cultivation of mature love.

Love is easy to say, but hard to define. Harry Stack Sullivan, MD, a great American psychiatrist, gave one of the best definitions we have heard. He defined love as a relationship in which one cares as much, or nearly as much , about the growth, development, welfare, and happiness of the beloved as one cares about one's own. Dyer defines love as a feeling of affection, together with giving to and serving the beloved, while expecting nothing in return. I think you will agree that this is a rigorous definition. It taxes one's spiritual development to have a powerful feeling of affection for another person, to give her whatever you can, serve her however you can and expect nothing in return.

Chopra defines love as the experience of oneness with the beloved. He wrote, "It is the realization that we are not just made of the same stuff; we *are* the same stuff." When, through meditation and discovery of your own true nature, you directly experience the oneness between you and all other life forms, then love comes naturally out of this consciousness. Even so, changing the old habits so that you give to and serve your beloved while expecting nothing in return takes hard practice and great spiritual discipline. The reward is a relationship that is rich in fulfillment, fun, creativity, and healing power—and remarkably short on fighting and frustration.

FOUR ADDITIONAL INGREDIENTS

Dyer proposes four additional ingredients for a loving relationship. These are:

1. Relinquish your need to be right. As Bob Dylan sang, "You're right from your side; I'm right from mine..." Chopra has observed that the mechanics of perception are such that it is inevitable that people see things differently and therefore have different perceptions of what is right. To let this be O.K. removes a tremendous obstacle to loving relationships.

Unfortunately, some people would rather be right than be happy!

2. Allow space. Gilbran in *The Prophet* said, "Be together; but let there be spaces in your togetherness, as the pillars of the temple stand apart and the cypress and the hemlock grow not in one another's shadow." Allowing those you love to have their own space when they want it and need it is to give the relationship room to grow, evolve, and renew itself. When our children were teenagers, it became clear to me that, if I were going to have the kind of adult/adult relationship with the children that I wanted, I would have to learn to love the children with an open hand. When the children were small, I tried to protect them and spare them what suffering I could. Now that they were maturing and growing up, the relationship had to change to a more mature one. I discovered that, if I held the children in an open hand—not clutching or trying to control—they were more likely to return to my "hand" for nurturing and companionship. Since I was brought up to be an "overfunctioning mother", this was a difficult but important part of backing off and allowing the children to grow into the person he/she wanted to be.

3. Eliminate the idea of ownership. Acknowledge that you do not own your beloved or your children, but that these relationships are a *gift* to be cherished and never coerced. Read the chapter on children in *The Prophet* by Gibran. He states, "Your children are not your children. They come through you but not from you...."

4. Know that you do not have to understand. Since each mind is unique, each understanding will be unique and there will be things that your beloved thinks, says, does, and feels that you will never understand. Do not make a problem out of it. You really do not have to understand!

Of all Dyer's wisdom about relationships, it seems to us that his emphasis on loving and serving without expecting anything in return is the most powerful. Adopting this attitude sets us free from a whole chain reaction of disappointment, anger, resentment, and broken relationships. Practicing this principle does not mean that we accept abuse from another person or become her slave. We may need to love and serve the other person from a safe distance, if she chooses to behave in an abusive or destructive way toward us. We will have to set limits on what we do for our beloved, although we love unconditionally. Limits are necessary to enable us to keep balance and harmony in our lives and to have time and energy to fulfill our missions.

EMPATHIC LISTENING

Another powerful principle for relationships that are long on fulfillment, short on frustration, and strongly contributory to the 100 year healthspan is, "Seek first to understand, then to be understood." Dr. Stephen Covey has eloquently articulated this in *The Seven Habits of Highly Effective People*. He gives an elegant, powerful, and useful system for doing so. He calls it "empathic listening". We encourage you to read what Covey has to say, or listen to him make his excellent presentation in his audiocassette album by the same title as the book. If you learn and practice empathic listening, as described by Covey, we guarantee that your human relationships, and particularly your intimate relationships, will improve dramatically.

Covey has one other recommendation that is so valuable that we will mention it here. That is, whenever you disagree with a person who is important to you, or disagree about a matter that is important to you, state the other person's position to that person's satisfaction before you state your disagreement. Of course, to do this you probably will have had to listen empathetically to the other person. Most people, including the two of us, find it hard to remember to do this when the disagreement is about a gut issue, but if you do it, the results are usually magical. Covey has some useful examples in the chapter I have cited.

THE IMPORTANCE OF COMMUNICATING POSITIVE EMOTIONS

Many of us who grew up during the depression had parents who needed to put most of their available energy into trying to keep food on the table and clothes on the backs of the members of the families. Working hard to supply material needs was the way that most males communicated to their families that they loved them. Most females communicated their love for the family members by cooking nourishing food and keeping the clothes cleaned and darned. There were all too few compliments and too little praise or feelings of love expressed. On the other hand, when someone had stepped out of line and had done something displeasing, punishment was oftentimes swift and severe.

John was standing at his father's hospital bed when his father died. Mother went over and put her arm around John and said, "You know, your father always loved you." John began to cry. Mother ran out into the hall and got a nurse to come in; after all, males do not cry. John said to them, "I am not crying because my father died; I am crying because he never told me that he loved me." Yes, it is important that we communicate to the significant people in our lives what is pleasing and displeasing to us; otherwise, they are left trying to read our minds as to what we want and need. Let us emphasize again the importance of communicating the positives in the relationship. Remember that what we keep our minds on expands in our lives. When we keep our thoughts and words on the positive aspects of the other person, those positive attributes will be the ones that will most likely be developed. Keep your mind and thoughts on the weaknesses of the other and those weaknesses will probably multiply.

While we were teaching this concept at one of the Elderhostels, one man shared the following story with the group. A farmer told his wife that he often looked at the beautiful land that she had helped him cultivate, and he often thought of how well she had done keeping nourishing food on the table, clothes cleaned, children well cared for. He said to her that, when he thought of all these blessings she had brought into his life, it took all he could do to keep from telling her how much he appreciated it and loved her!

Regularly telling the important people in your life that you appreciate them, that you love them is a habit that I would like for us all to cultivate. Do not wait until someone is dying!

All family members are healthier emotionally when positive feelings are regularly shared. Try giving at least 10 compliments (called warm fuzzies in Transactional Analysis) each day to see what happens. Most of us feel so much better when we have conveyed positive emotions to others, and we usually get many warm fuzzies for ourselves when we open the lines of communication to express, in words and action, appreciation for what we too often take for granted.

Marriage is perhaps the biggest guessing game in the world. The myth for years has been that, if you love me, you would know what I want/need without my having to ask for it. That myth has now been thoroughly debunked. Learn to ask for what you want! The fact that I ask for something that I need/want does not guarantee that I will get it, but it does make it more likely.

There is one final golden key to relationships that are so good that they make you want to stay healthy, vigorous, and vital for 100 years to enjoy them. It is the concept that every person you meet has some truth that you need for your spiritual evolution and you have some truth the other person needs for his or hers. James Redfield in *The Celestine Prophecy* describes this in the eighth insight, "The New Interpersonal Ethic." There is something magical about approaching each encounter with this attitude. Redfield describes a powerful technology for facilitating this exchange of vital information. He tells you how to connect with nature in a way that builds your energy by tapping into the ultimate energy source of the universe. Then, when you are full of energy, you spontaneously experience a loving attitude toward others and project energy to the other person in a way that Redfield clearly describes. This energizes the other person to speak the truth she has for you in the clearest and most effective way. This then energizes you to reciprocate.

Redfield tells how to select those with whom you should establish the contact that permits this exchange of information. Of course, you can not do this with everybody: it takes time and energy, so you need to know which people are more important for opening this kind of communication. Redfield says that if the other person looks familiar but you have actually never met her, or if there is spontaneous eye contact, this person is particularly likely to have important information for you, and you for her. He encourages initiating conversation, when it is appropriate and feasible. This technology is clearly described in *The Celestine Prophecy* and its accompanying experiential guide. It is on the *must* reading list for the attainment of the 100-year healthspan.

CONCLUSION

I cannot tell you how much your relationships will improve and how much satisfaction and joy they will bring into your life and the lives of others if you will learn and regularly use the wisdom of these three great teachers. We consider the following ideas to be the most potent. Dyer: Love means to give to and serve your beloved while expecting nothing in return. Covey: Seek first to understand, then to be understood. Use empathic listening when there is an important disagreement. State the other person's position to her satisfaction before stating your disagreement. Redfield: Every person you meet has truth that you need for your spiritual evolution and you have truth they need for theirs. Establish contact with the more important of these people and give the other person energy from your own inexhaustible supply, so that she may speak her truth as clearly as possible to you. Then, to the best of your ability, give her the truth you have for her.

We are in the early stages of a revolution in human relationships. Part of this revolution will be an emphasis on each person empowering others to move toward their full physical, mental, spiritual, and economic potential. The old paradigm was power over others; the new one is empowering others. As you participate in this revolution, you become one of the human beings necessary to create the critical mass that will result in this quality of relationships becoming the norm for our society. Your resulting fulfillment and joy will contribute in a major way to your claiming and enjoying your natural birthright.

The simplest way that I can summarize creative relationships is this: treat your significant other and your children the same way that you would treat your best friend. Do not say anything negative to them that you would not say to your friend. Creative relationships must take place in an atmosphere of mutual respect.

Integrity is discerning the right thing, doing it, and openly saying why.

—Author unknown

Chapter 11

BUILDING and BALANCING ENERGY

ENERGY MATTERS
Quantum physics teaches us that energy becomes matter.
The Vedas teach us that energy precedes matter.
Energy medicine teaches us that energy controls matter.
We may conclude, therefore, that energy matters.
—OJW

INTRODUCTION

Energy is defined as the ability to do work. The work under consideration in this chapter is all of the transformations that go on in the Whole Self as you live and function. One kind of energy is called subtle energy because it can be measured only by the most sensitive instruments, detected subjectively, or recognized by its effects. It is the kind of energy that healers transfer to their patients, often through their hands, but sometimes through the focusing of attention without physical contact.

In one well-known experiment, a healer held some seeds in his hands. Then the seeds were planted adjacent to other seeds from the same package that had not been in the healer's hands. Someone, who did not know which seeds had been "treated" and which had not, then evaluated the growth of the seedlings. The treated seeds clearly outgrew the others. A similar experiment was done without treating the seeds but watering one group of seedlings with water that had been in a container held in the healer's hands. The other seedlings were watered from the same source but without the water's being in the healer's hands. Again, the seedlings that were watered with the treated water were judged by evaluators, who did not know which was which, to outperform the others. Therefore, we are talking about a subtle energy that is necessary for all transformations that go on in the Whole Self and, obviously, in other life forms as well.

In a conversation with Dr. Roy Curtain, the physicist whose experiments with a random number generator were described in Chapter Three, I asked Roy if my college physics knowledge was still up to date to the extent that matter and energy are the fundamental components of the Universe. Roy replied, "Matter, energy—and intelligence."

Therefore, I learned that something new had been added to the Universe since I took college physics. Roy defined intelligence as "that which decides." As previously mentioned, energy is the ability to do work. Therefore, when the intelligence of the Universe decides what to do, energy is the ability to do it: produce matter, for example. Quantum physicists have worked out the mathematical formulas that define the process by which energy produces matter. This process is called super-string theory; interesting, but beyond the scope of this discussion. What is of practical importance here is that since energy is necessary for all transformations that go on in the Whole Self, some of it is necessary to sustain life. In order to sustain health, enough of it is necessary—and it must be balanced. In this chapter, we will consider both of these issues: how to have enough energy and how to keep it sufficiently balanced.

An old recipe for rabbit stew begins, *"First you have to get a rabbit."* Let us consider the process of getting energy. It helps to know where to go to get it. The Field of Pure Consciousness, the higher part of the Higher Self, is the inexhaustible reservoir of energy. Whenever a person focuses attention in the Field of Pure Consciousness, he taps into this reservoir and the energy level in his Whole Self increases. That is why, the first time I did zazen, after only five minutes I felt increased energy. Those people who regularly access quiet alertness for twenty or thirty minutes twice daily regularly replenish their energy supply. They consistently have substantially more energy than would be the case if they were not tapping into the energy of the Field of Pure Consciousness. Even accessing quiet alertness, which is the gateway to the Field of Pure Consciousness, once a day will increase energy. That is not as satisfactory as twice a day for the same reason that eating one meal a day does not maintain strength all day as well as eating two. When one is under heavy stress, the experience of quiet alertness three times a day works even better. Eventually, when the power of attention is strong enough, awareness of the Field of Pure Consciousness is continuous, even when one is intensely involved in activities. This provides a continuous input of new energy, the ideal situation for enjoying abundant energy.

There are other ways of accessing energy. James Redfield describes an effective and enjoyable technology in *The Celestine Prophecy*. The approach he recommends is to focus attention on some object of natural beauty, such as a huge old tree or a flower. If attention is focused long enough and strongly enough, eventually the object will appear to glow. That indicates a transfer of energy from nature to the Whole Self. Whenever one is low on energy, Redfield recommends this procedure for replenishing. "Eat before you get hungry," is a wise recommendation from Dr. Barry Sears, in his best seller, *The Zone*. We recommend the same approach for energy: regularly replete energy before you feel yourself running low on it.

Another good, simple way to rebuild energy is to walk on the earth. The earth has tremendous energy, which you can access by walking on the earth. You can gain energy if you walk on pavement, but the process is less efficient. If you can do your walking in a high-energy place, such as along a stream, around a lake, or on the beach, the process is substantially enhanced. It does not take a lot of walking: twenty or thirty minutes for most people will produce a valuable energy increase. Not only does walking increase energy, but it helps to balance it throughout the Whole Self. This double benefit of walking is probably an important part of the many health benefits gained through this activity.

THE FLICK PROTOCOL

The most powerful energy building and balancing procedure that we know is the Flick Protocol. If you do only one intervention on the energy level of your Whole Self, we recommend this one. Bart Flick, MD, an orthopedic surgeon and primary researcher in wound healing and tissue regeneration, developed it. The Protocol is an integration of four energy enhancing techniques. Each is valuable separately. The synergy of the integration of the four is uniquely effective in creating the quantity, quality and balance of energy necessary for optimum well-being, effectiveness, and zest for life every day—and for the 100-year healthspan.

Benefits include:

- **Increased energy and stamina.** When I am so tired that I doubt that I can do the Protocol, but do it anyway, I get a surge of energy that is good for another hour or two of work—or play.

- **Increased feeling of well-being, self-confidence, and freedom.** Some people will get at least as much endorphin rush from doing the Protocol as from jogging three miles. Many will experience a delightful freedom of movement and comfort and enjoyment of their bodies. These are fundamental factors in quality of life.

- **Accelerated healing of injury and disease.** This is important for everyone. It is critically important for those who have serious, chronic, and/or life-threatening disease. Recovery depends largely on sufficient activation of the self-healing mechanism of the body. This Protocol is the most cost-effective, time-efficient, easiest way we know to accomplish this on the energy level. For some, it can mean the difference between life and death. For many, it will mean the difference between a predominance of comfort or discomfort. Dr. Flick told us of one of his patients who was in pain and about to have surgery for a large, bulging, intervertebral disc. After nine months using one component of the Protocol, The Five Rites of Rejuvenation, the patient had no symptoms—and no surgery.

- **Reversal of biological age.** We have observed improved flexibility and balance, regrowth of hair on a bald head, darkening of gray hair, and smoothing of skin and wrinkles. A patient of ours was pleased to report enhanced sexual potency.

- **Decreased need for sleep**, often one to two hours less.

- **Cost-effectiveness:** We know of nothing else that improves so much with so little time and effort. The Protocol combines the benefits of yoga, meditation, and calisthenics—and delivers these benefits and more in a fraction of the time it would take to do the three things separately.

The components of the Protocol are

- A chi gong practice
- The Five Rites of Rejuvenation
- Yoga fire breath
- The Denny Johnson Protocol for Clearing the Family-Tree

Chi gong

- Place a clock with a sweep second hand where you can see it easily without turning your head.

- Stand erect, and then bend your knees until you can no longer see your feet. Hold this position throughout the procedure. See illustration on page 248.

- Hold your arms at your sides. Bend your elbows so that your forearms are at right angles to your arms with hands pointed forward, palms down, fingers together, thumbs against sides of palms.

- Bend your index fingers at right angles at the first joint away from the knuckles.

- Hold this position for 30 seconds. If 30 seconds is easy, start with one minute.

- Straighten your index finger. Bend your second finger at right angles at the first joint away from the knuckle. Hold this position for 30 seconds. Straighten your second finger. Follow the same procedure with your fourth and fifth fingers.

- As your strength and stamina increase, add 30 to 60 seconds at a time to each position until you are doing each one for three minutes. Adding 30 seconds per week to each position is good, but vary that to do what feels right for you. The full procedure takes 12 minutes. You are unlikely to find anything else that improves your quality and quantity of energy so much in such a short time.

- *You can multiply the benefits by doing this practice as a meditation.* To do this, focus your attention on what you are doing with your body and with your breath as you breathe normally through your nose. When thoughts come into your mind, immediately refocus your attention on your body and your breath. It is easier and more effective to do this in a quiet place, while looking at a natural object such as a plant, a tree, or a landscape. Close your eyes if you need to reduce visual distractions.

Here is the special meditation I mentioned in Chapter 8, in the section on sabotaging the ego. I encourage you to try it, because you are likely to be delighted with the experience. Wait until you have learned the chi gong procedure: do not try too many new things at once!

- During the time you keep your index finger bent, practice bringing the feeling of love into your awareness of your Higher Power. Hold both together in your awareness. If

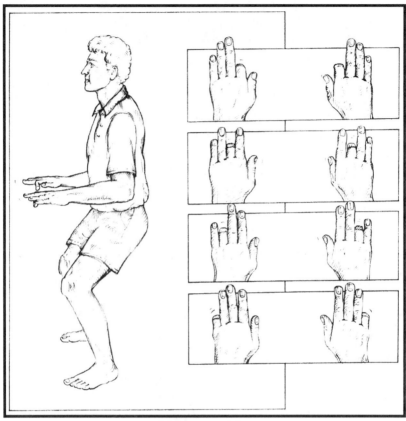

Chi Gong Positions

you have a picture or a symbol for your Higher Power, it may help to look at it.

- During second finger time, with each inhalation silently think the name of your Higher Power. On the exhalation, think of something for which you are grateful. Feel the gratitude to your Higher Power for that blessing or grace in your life.

- During third finger time, focus your attention on feeling the energy and the spiritual presence of your Higher Power.

- Fourth finger: open your awareness to knowing what your Higher Power has for you to do today. It is natural to want to serve and please your Higher Power, when you feel deep love and intense gratitude.

You are likely to have some powerful, thrilling, and beneficial experiences if you persist in this practice for a month or two. The energy and intelligence of your Higher Power will flow through you increasingly and manifest in the world. You become a blessing to others and to the world in ways you cannot even imagine.

After you have been doing this for a few weeks you will probably enjoy the results so much that you may want to add another session each day, doing one morning and evening.

The Five Rites of Rejuvenation

The Five Rites are unique in our experience. We do not even know how to classify them. They integrate characteristics of yoga, chakra (energy) balancing and tuning, calisthenics, and meditation. In "Strengthening the Power of Attention" Genevieve described four paths of meditation: body, intellect, action and emotions. The Five Rites combine the first three.

The Eye of Revelation, by Peter Kelder, tells the interesting story of how The Five Rites came from Tibet to England and then to the US. The book was copyrighted in 1939, but the knowledge is still not in general use. That such a powerful technology has been generally ignored for nearly 60 years is as surprising as the neglect of the Maharishi Effect, described in "The Power of Attention." I believe the reasons are similar: the level of awareness in our culture was insufficient to enable enough people to appreciate the value of either technology. Until about 16% of a population adopt a new idea, the "hundredth-monkey phenomenon" does not work and the new concept fails to come into general use. Probably, by now, the awareness of enough people has reached a level that can appreciate the value of both of these technologies and put the hundredth monkey to work. When that happens, our whole culture will pull up to a significantly higher level of health and happiness. One of the joys of writing this book is spreading the word of these two powerful, neglected blessings.

The Five Rites are surprisingly, unexpectedly, powerful. Like any other powerful thing, they must be used skillfully for maximum benefit with minimum risk. There is a Zen saying, "A blade of grass held unskillfully can cut the hand." Potential risks in doing The Five Rites unskillfully include joint and/or muscle injury, overstimulation, fatigue, and failure to gain full benefit. The last risk is the most dangerous because it can lead to discouragement and abandonment of a practice that would be a major asset in increasing your quality and quantity of life. Chopra says it well, "Adding years to your life and life to your years."

For skillful use of The Five Rites:

- Read *The Eye of Revelation* and watch the video, *The Five Rites of Rejuvenation,* before you begin. Each document has critical information not available in the other. The book gives instructions on how many repetitions of each Rite to start with and how to increase to the full number of repetitions. Because of the power of The Five Rites, it is important not to overdo them. The video shows correct technique that is essential to gaining full benefit. The diagrams in the book cannot do this adequately.

- Follow the directions carefully and precisely.

- Consult your healthcare professional before beginning, if you have bone or joint problems or any serious medical condition.

- Do not strain to do any of the Rites. Follow directions in the book and video on how to do them without strain. Pay particular attention to the instructions in the book on how to start and gradually increase the number of repetitions of each Rite until you reach the full count. The video is ambiguous, the book is clear: do one repetition of each Rite three times a day for one week. Then do two repetitions once a day. After three or four days, do three repetitions once a day. Add two repetitions each week until you are doing the full count of 21 once a day. Then, if you wish to gain additional benefit, start a second session each day. Begin the second session with two repetitions and increase as before. If it is easy to increase repetitions faster than this and you want faster results, it is permissible to do so. Be alert for fatigue, overstimulation, or pain: they warn that you are increasing repetitions too fast. The saying, "No pain, no gain" may be true if you are training for the Olympics. When you are training for the 100-year healthspan, it is "No pain, no gain—no brain."

See the Resources section of the Appendix for where to get the book and video.

Yoga fire breath

This is also called bellows breath. Andrew Weil, M.D., calls it the stimulating breath. Whatever you call it, it is a valuable way to gain energy. After completing each Rite, stand with hands on hips and do this breath technique for one minute.

1. Touch the tip of your tongue to the place where your gum and upper teeth meet. Keep it there throughout the minute.

2. Breathe rapidly through your nose, keeping your mouth lightly closed. Your inhalations and exhalations should be of equal length and as short as possible (as many as three cycles per second, if you can do that comfortably). You should feel muscular effort at the base of your neck, just above your collarbones, and in your diaphragm (try putting your hands on these spots to get a sense of movement).

3. Start with 15 seconds, and then breathe normally for the other 45 seconds. Gradually increase the time by 5 seconds, as you get comfortable with the procedure, until you are doing it for a full minute.

Focus attention on the feeling created by air rushing in and out through your nostrils. Some students of subtle energy believe that the rapid flow of large volumes of air over the deeper nasal membranes stimulates the release of endorphins. Endorphins are powerful messenger molecules that strengthen immune function and produce the experience of exhilaration and well-being.

The Denny Ray Johnson Protocol for Clearing for the Family Tree

Denny Johnson is a gifted naturopath who appreciates the power of the spoken word. As Chopra says in *Sacred Verses, Healing Sounds*, "Words send messages to the core of cellular life." Johnson has devised a system for using words to remove the toxic, discordant energy patterns that have been passed down in families for generations, and replacing it with harmonious energy. Replacing discordant energy with harmonious energy permits, as Johnson puts it, "...the engagement and expression of the genetic blueprint of perfection throughout all vibrational levels of the mind and body of the individual and the entire family tree."

Since this is a new concept, most people will not use it, but most of those who have report extraordinary experiences of healing and higher functioning in their families. A patient recently told me that members of her extended family began communicating with one another within days after she did the protocol. Communication had been cut off for years.

The protocol is in Appendix 1.

Relative Power of the Components of the Flick Protocol

Since it takes about 30 minutes to do the Flick Protocol, exclusive of Clearing the Family Tree, you may be interested in what the relative benefit of each component is and how much time it takes. If you do not choose to commit half an hour of your day right away, it is possible to spend less time and still gain major benefit. As your energy, mental clarity, experience of well being, and productivity improve, you will be accomplishing more in less time. You may then decide to invest some of the time you have saved in adding more components and multiplying the benefit. The following estimates are based on our experience with the protocol.

- **The Five Rites**. It takes about 13 minutes to do 21 repetitions of each rite. The Five Rites contribute about 50% of the total benefit

- **Chi gong** takes 12 minutes and contributes about 20%.

- **Fire breath** takes five minutes and contributes 10%

- **Clearing for the Family Tree** takes 30 minutes once or twice a month and contributes 20%. If you do one clearing per month, the average daily time expenditure is one minute per day. This makes this component the most time-efficient, but you may need to rest the day after each clearing and you probably will not be as efficient and productive as usual for two or three days. During the rest of the month, you will probably more than make up for the lost time.

The synergy of the components is surprisingly powerful. The effect of the complete protocol is far greater than the sum of its parts: 1+1+1+1= a lot more than 4! As you add each component, notice how the value escalates.

Tactics and times for getting started

You can start with minimal time expenditure. You can do one repetition of each Rite in less than five minutes. If you start with one minute in each of the four chi gong positions, that is four minutes; so you can get started in less than 10 minutes three times a day for the first week. In the second week, the time expenditure actually decreases, since you will be doing the Protocol only once a day. Two repetitions of each Rite take about 10 minutes; two minutes of each chi gong position require eight minutes. Therefore, you are spending 18 minutes per day instead of thirty. You could add Fire Breath between each of the Rites, spend another five minutes on the Protocol, multiply the benefit, and still be investing less than 30 minutes per day. From then on, your increased productivity, well-being, energy, clarity, zest for life, and decreased need for sleep will more than compensate you for the time you invest.

The decreased need for sleep may, by itself, result in a net time gain for you. You will probably need one to two hours less sleep in each 24-hour cycle. If you need even one hour less sleep, that will permit you to invest 30 minutes twice a day to do the full Flick Protocol with *no* loss of time from your usual schedule—and all of the benefits about which you have just been reading. This is about as close as anybody gets to having his or her cake and eating it too. A word of caution: most people get too little sleep. This is one of the abusive lifestyles discussed in Chapter Two. If you do not recall that discussion, please review it—very important. If you are already sleep-deprived, do the Protocol, keep on sleeping the same number of hours, and suffer less cumulative damage—maybe none at all—because you need less sleep than previously.

Now is the best time to start. When I was a boy and Mother told me to do something, I sometimes protested, " I don't know how."

She often replied, "Well, you won't learn any younger." You can start now and not get too much older before you learn—and earn splendid benefits.

Suggestion:

- Order the Five Rites book and video from one of the sources listed in the Resources section of the Appendix.

- Begin doing the chi gong practice today. By the time the materials you have ordered arrive, you will already have more energy for doing the other components of the Protocol.

You now have our pick for the premier intervention for energy building and balancing. If you do only one of these things, your energy and your Whole Self will say, "Thanks, I needed that!" If you do them all, you will probably look at your quality of life and say, "Wow! Something sure happened!" When we skip the Protocol, we notice a decrease in the quality of our lives. We miss the quality until we do the Protocol again—so we do not skip it often. Once you start to enjoy the enhanced way you feel and function, we do not think you will either.

BRING ON THE BIOCHEMISTRY!

In addition to these behavioral means of gaining energy, there are a couple of biochemical interventions that often work well as a rescue remedy, while you are waiting for the behavioral practices to become fully effective. We will make a more comprehensive presentation on nutritional supplementation in the next chapter. For now, I am assuming that you will be taking one of the Basic Preventive multiple vitamin formulas and at least 6 grams of vitamin C a day. For people who have not been using this combination, starting it will usually produce a significant energy gain.

If you are already doing this and are still short on energy, you could add Coenzyme-Q-10. This remarkable nutrient improves the efficiency of electron transfer in the mitochondria. Mitochondria are the structures in every cell of your body that act as tiny furnaces, burning sugar and oxygen to energy and carbon dioxide. A lot of things, including environmental toxins and severe infections, as well as free radical activity from other sources, injure the DNA in mitochondria. The result is loss of efficiency that is sometimes severe and incapacitating. Chronic fatigue syndrome is an extreme example, but many people have this problem to a lesser degree. Coenzyme-Q-10 increases the efficiency of electron transfer in the mitochondria, usually producing gratifying improvements in energy. Seventy-five milligrams twice a day is a good starting dose, although some people may need to take 100 or 150 milligrams twice daily for full response. Some people may respond to as little as 30 milligrams twice daily.

Co-Q-10 is a wonderful substance. Its only disadvantage is that it is relatively expensive. However, if you are severely short on energy, it can serve you well as a rescue remedy for two or three months while you are using more cost-effective behavioral interventions to attain an abundant energy supply. Since Co-Q-10 is expensive and hard to absorb, use the chewable tablets and take it with a little fat to improve absorption. Two or three almonds, half a dozen peanuts, or half a teaspoon of olive oil, flax oil, or two capsules of fish oil concentrate will be enough, or take it with meals.

Another nutritional supplement that is useful in energy enhancement is alpha lipoic acid. This substance protects mitochondrial DNA against free radical damage. If you use a combination of alpha lipoic acid and Co-Q-10, you are enhancing the efficiency of your mitochondria, while at the same time protecting them against further damage. Alpha lipoic acid 100 milligrams three times daily will probably work well for most people. Since alpha lipoic acid improves insulin sensitivity, diabetics should monitor blood sugar levels closely when they start taking it. Reduction in insulin may be needed.

BALANCING ENERGY

Once you get the rabbit, you need to make the stew. In energy terms, making the stew means balancing your available energy. Here are some methods for doing it.

Labyrinths

In addition to walking on the earth, there are other ways to balance energy and keep it balanced. One of these is to regularly walk through a labyrinth. A labyrinth is an ancient geometric form, usually consisting of eight concentric circles outlined on the earth with stone or plants. There are openings in the circles permitting one to pass from one circle to the next. The labyrinth was designed to both balance energy and expand awareness. A labyrinth should be built where the earth energies are favorable to it. A dowser skilled in labyrinth construction knows how to locate these favorable places. One of our friends, Richard Cottrell, is a labyrinth builder. We were fortunate that he located and out-lined a labyrinth for us at our home, Questing Wode. Part of our daily routine is to walk through the labyrinth. At the entrance, we ask the question, "What must I do today for maximum mis-sion fulfillment?" As we walk the first circle in the labyrinth the question is, "What thoughts come to mind about this question?" In the second circle, "How do I feel about the thoughts that came to mind?" In the third circle, "What are the physical aspects of this question?" In the fourth circle, "What are the spiritual as-pects of this question?" In the fifth circle we feel and express our gratitude to the Field of Pure Consciousness. In the sixth and seventh circles, we put attention on forming a vision of what we must do that day for maximum mission fulfillment. That brings us to the eighth circle, which is the center of the labyrinth. There, we spend some time affirming the happiness of fulfillment that comes from the process of accomplishing our missions. We also mentally send some of the energy and information of The Field of Pure Consciousness, the energy of Questing Wode, and the energy of our love to family members, friends, patients, and all beings.

After leaving the center of the labyrinth, we re-trace the cir-cles in reverse order. In the seventh and sixth circles, attention goes to further clarifying the vision of what to do that day. In the fifth, we give thanks to the Field of Pure Consciousness. In the fourth, we consider the spiritual implications of the vision for the day. In the third, the consideration is of the physical implica-tions; in the second, the emotional implications, and in the first circle, we notice what our thoughts are about the vision for the day. At the mouth of the labyrinth we stop and thank the laby-rinth, Richard Cottrell, who designed it, and all those beings who have brought this knowledge of the energy-and-awareness-enhancing effects of labyrinths down through the ages. We have reason to give thanks. We always come out of the labyrinth with a much better understanding of what we must do that day and with enhanced energy for doing it. We usually come out with a feeling of bliss, even when we went in feeling over-whelmed, anxious, angry, or confused.

Even without the favorable earth energies, the labyrinth pattern is well worth walking. Some churches have painted the labyrinth pattern on canvas, which they unroll in a large open space in the church, making the technology available for worshipers who wish to experience enhanced energy, balance, and mental and spiritual clarity. When we are out of town, I will sometimes find an open, grassy place and walk the labyrinth pattern there. I am pleased to say that I have not yet been arrested for this bizarre behavior. I do try to be discreet about it and not do it when there are a lot of other people around.

Not long ago, I experienced the healing power of energy balancing in the labyrinth. At that time, my energy was sufficiently out of balance that I had a plantar wart on the ball of my right foot and an infected callus on the heel of the left. Every step was painful enough to make me think about whom I could get to tend the garden when I became unable to walk. I hobbled into the labyrinth and did the protocol as just described. I was not even thinking about healing. As I stood at the center of the labyrinth, doing the affirmation, both feet started to tingle. I knew immediately that healing was taking place through energy balancing. Richard had done his work well. The coherent energy of the labyrinth was strong enough to shift the energy of my Whole Self in the direction of health. Within seconds, the pain in my feet began to subside; within minutes, I was walking comfortably.

For more information on labyrinth technology for energy enhancement, see *Labyrinths: Ancient Myths and Modern Uses*, by Sig Lonegren.

Getting help from others

So far, we have been considering things you can do for yourself to balance energy. Another option is to get someone to help you with it. In the last five years, there has been a proliferation of methods and a great increase of number of practitioners offering this service. Some of the more widely known and practiced systems for assisted energy balancing are Therapeutic Touch, acupuncture, acupressure, and Reiki. All of these systems are extremely operator-dependent. Any of them, in the hands of a skilled, spiritually developed, conscientious practitioner can yield good-to-excellent results. Any of them, in the hands of someone who is not skilled, spiritually developed, and competent in the procedure, can lead to results that are at best only marginally helpful, and at worst, harmful. We discussed some of the mechanics of this in the chapter on The Power of Attention. Selecting the right practitioner can be challenging, and is certainly important.

Licensure and certification probably will not help much, although it does not hurt. Your best bet is probably to select a practitioner who uses a method that is intuitively comfortable to you, and then interview the practitioner. If your intuition tells you that you and this individual are likely to be able to work well together, then you might decide to have a treatment session. Notice how you feel afterward, particularly several days afterwards. If you were not comfortable with the procedure, that is a warning flag; but if several days later you feel better than usual and can not account for it any other way, you may have found someone who can be of substantial help to you.

These energy-balancing procedures can be powerful enough to stir up unpleasant sensations and experiences. It is somewhat like having surgery. After major surgery you will not feel so well the next day; but once the pain subsides, you may be glad for the next thirty or forty years that you had the procedure done. If this sort of thing happens with energy balancing, you are probably in the hands of a good practitioner. However, if you feel worse immediately afterwards and no better several days later, it might be well to look further.

Choosing the right practitioner may not be as hard as it sounds, because the more time you spend in quiet alertness and the more attention you pay to your Higher Self, the sharper and more accurate your intuition becomes. Eventually you will know right away whether a particular person is the right one to help you with energy balancing. In the early stages of your adventure, however, caution is advisable. As Thomas Jefferson said, "Delay is preferable to error."

Part of keeping energy balanced is knowing where your energy is going. Many people "leak" energy without being aware of it. For those having energy balance problems, we recommend the audiotape album, *Energy Anatomy,* by Caroline Myss, Ph.D. Myss describes a way of monitoring energy dynamics and getting more control over them. She calls it "energy accounting."

Remember Redfield's statement, "Where attention goes energy flows." When energy is going where you do not want it to go, you can focus attention on what is happening. That brings to your awareness where your energy is going. By refocusing attention where you do want your energy to go, you redirect it. This is an important step toward energy balancing. With energy balanced, you are in a strong position to balance your biochemistry. The next chapter gives you information about how to do that important process.

Stand with anybody that stands right—and part with him when he goes wrong.

—Abraham Lincoln

Chapter 12

BALANCING BIOCHEMISTRY

INTRODUCTION

Biochemistry means, "Life chemistry, or the chemistry of life." There are various estimates of how many chemical reactions are going on in your body all the time in order for you to be alive. The one that seems most likely is 4,000 to 5,000. That is a lot of biochemistry, and it all has to be well balanced in order for you to have your best shot at the 100-year healthspan. It has to be fairly well balanced for you to stay in this existence at all. A little too far out of balance and you are off on Justice Holmes' "...great adventure!"

As you know by now, there are a lot of things in modern life that can jerk your biochemistry out of balance. Fortunately, there are also a lot of things you can do to keep it balanced, in addition to balancing your consciousness, which you already know about. You are about to learn some of the other important things for balancing biochemistry.

SLEEP

This may be a surprise—if you do not recall the list of Dream Destroyers in Chapter 2. Surveys have repeatedly shown that most people in our culture do not get enough sleep. There are several reasons. The most powerful is that most people do not get paid or praised for sleeping. Another reason is that most people do not know how much sleep they need. People vary greatly in their sleep requirements. Ayurveda recognizes a constitutional type called *vata* that may need as little as four hours sleep in 24. Another type, *kapha*, may need 10 hours. Another reason is that awareness of sleep need gets distorted by substances such as sedatives and stimulants— and by alarm clocks. Whatever the need for sleep, meeting it is essential to biochemical balance. Maintaining that balance in a constantly changing environment takes energy that is available only during sleep. The body, according to ayurveda, goes through an important, energy-intensive, self-cleansing cycle between 10 PM and 2 AM. If you are not asleep during those hours, the process is underpowered and inefficient. Over time, toxicity builds up. The modern science of cell physiology has estimated that 90% of the energy used by each cell goes for maintenance and repair. That much energy is available only during sleep—and meditation. This raises the interesting question, "Can meditation substitute for sleep?" The answer is, "To a degree, but not completely." People who begin to meditate regularly often find that they need about one hour less sleep than they did before.

Since sleep is so important, how can you tell when you are getting enough? Simple:

1. Avoid the routine use of sedatives and avoid stimulants such as caffeine, ephedra, and guarana. These substances override the natural wisdom of the body. Using them is like turning your headlights off while driving at night because you do not like the looks of the road.

2. Turn off your alarm clock. When you start waking up when you need to get up and you do not doze off when you get still during the day, you are probably getting enough sleep.

Actually, it is not quite that simple. If you are depressed, you may feel a need to sleep more than you really need to. Alternatively, you may wake up much too early, be unable to go back to sleep, and them have to fight sleep all day. The imbalances creating the depression have to be corrected before you know what your natural need for sleep is. If you hate your job or whatever it is you are waking up to do, this may have a distorting effect on sleeping and waking. If this is an issue, it urgently needs to be addressed, because few things shorten the healthspan so much as hating one's job. That is why more heart attacks happen at nine o'clock on Monday morning than at any other hour in the week.

Although it is not foolproof, the alarm clock test is worth trying. It can tell you more than your need for sleep, important as that is. Bob Dylan sang, "...a false clock tries to tick out my time/ to disgrace, distract and bother me..." Your true clock is somewhere in your Whole Self, not on the table by your bed. Do not let a false clock tick out your time. If you do, you will run out of time before you run out of 100-year healthspan!

WATER

Next, we will consider water, because most of those four or five thousand biochemical reactions that go on in your body all the time depend on water. Too much water or too little water and they do not go very well. When they do not go very well, you do not go very well. When there is a water imbalance, it is usually too little, not too much. For optimum biochemical balance, you have to be drinking at least two quarts of water every twenty-four hours. If you are sweating a lot, it has to be more than that.

Most people do not even come close to drinking two quarts of water a day. Two quarts of fluid, maybe, but other kinds of fluid do not balance biochemistry very well and may actually be a serious imbalancing factor. Therefore, it has to be water, and reasonably pure. As you know after reading the Dream Destroyers chapter, pure water is hard to find, and probably cannot be had out of the tap fed by a municipal water system. In fact, the chemical taste of most water that comes out of taps from municipal systems is one reason that water has fallen out of favor as a beverage. Of course, the billions of dollars beverage companies spend convincing you that, if you will just drink their product, you will be swiftly wafted away to nirvana, tends to make people forget about water. However, when they do happen to think about it and what comes out of the tap smells and tastes as though it was drawn from the footbath at the "Y", it gets easier to believe the advertising hype about other liquids.

Pure water, on the other hand, tastes good. Since it tastes good and is essential to your biochemical balance, which is essential to your best chance for a 100-year healthspan, we need to consider how to get some. There are several options. One is to trust what comes out of the tap. If you are the type who buys big bridges from strangers in large cities, you probably will be comfortable with this one. Otherwise, you may want to go to option two, which is, buy distilled water. When you buy any kind of bottled water, you have to hope the person who slapped the label on the jug was honest. Some are, some are not. Even the honest ones sometimes make mistakes. The contamination of Perrier with benzene is an example. However, with distilled water you are probably better off than you are with tap water. You will not get the minerals that support health, but you can get them from your supplements. Bottled water in plastic containers tends to leach toxic chemicals out of the plastic, but even so, you are still probably better off than with tapwater.

Option three is to put a good filtration system into your kitchen plumbing. As water contamination gets worse, filtration systems get better. I think that we are at least holding our own and maybe gaining a little ground. The technology is advancing so fast that anything I write about today will be obsolete, or at least obsolescent, by the time you read this. Your best bet is, when you are ready to invest in a filtration system, to get consultation with a good environmental engineer. The salesperson at K-Mart or Home Depot (if you can find a salesperson) is not a reliable source of information about water filters. A person selling only one brand of water filter may be prejudiced in favor of that brand. An environmental engineer has access to a number of different filters and is in a stronger position to make an impartial choice. There are not a lot of environmental engineers around. The chance that you will find one at your local health department is vanishingly remote. If you live in a large city, you may be able to find an environmental engineer by looking in the Yellow Pages. In the Resources section of the Appendix, I have listed the name and phone number of a source for the water filtration system recommended by Julian Whitaker, M.D., editor of *the Health and Healing Newsletter.*

If your water comes from a well, deep or surface, testing is important. Most, if not all, surface water in the U.S. is contaminated with chemicals, but some of the deeper aquifers are still pure. Water testing will tell whether a particular well is drawing from one of these aquifers. *Warning: do not assume that water testing done by health departments will detect chemical contamination.* Those tests usually are for disease causing microorganisms only and for only a limited number of those. A positive health department test tells you that you have a problem, but a negative does not tell you that you do not have a problem. Contact information for a company who does water testing is in the Resources section.

Once you are drinking at least two quarts of pure water every day, you have taken an important step toward balancing your biochemistry. You probably will notice that you are already feeling better. The next step is the most powerful one: balancing biochemistry with nutrition.

FOOD

Hippocrates, the father of medicine, said, "Let your food be your medicine and your medicine your food." He was right, but if he said how to do it, the instructions got lost. We have had to wait 2500 years to find out how to do it. The first breakthrough came in the early 80's when medical researchers discovered powerful tissue hormones called eicosanoids. You will be hearing more about eicosanoids before you finish this book, but I can tell you now that they micromanage most of your biochemistry. If you get them balanced, they automatically balance much of the rest of your biochemistry. That is one way of getting hold of the kudzu root that I am always looking for because it lets you "...shake the whole State." In other words, I keep looking for one thing you can do that improves many things that grow out of the one thing, the way kudzu vines grow out of kudzu roots. For those who are not familiar with kudzu, I will say that kudzu grows very fast and will grow over everything around it. You can cut the kudzu vines back to the ground, but if you do not get rid of the roots, they will be back in an astonishingly short time.

The Zone

In 1995, the second breakthrough occurred that enabled me, and now you, to get hold of the nutritional kudzu root. In that year, Barry Sears, Ph.D. published *The Zone*. Sears, over a period of about ten years, worked out a way to use macronutrients (protein, fat, and carbohydrate) to balance eicosanoids. When I began to use this system for myself, and soon after for my patients, I found it the most powerful nutritional intervention of the many I have used in forty years of medical practice.

Four days after I began the Zone program, I was astonished to notice one morning that my lower back was no longer sore. I have a congenital deformity of two vertebrae in my lumbar spine. This created a favorable condition for arthritis, which set up years ago. My low back had been sore and stiff for as long as I can remember. It became noticeably better in 1976 when I began to meditate, but the soreness and stiffness did not completely go away. That morning, four days after I began the Zone program, there was no soreness or stiffness! I was impressed. The next day I noticed that my tennis elbow was definitely less tender and painful. I had endured it for nearly three months without any sign of improvement before that day. Within another ten days, it was completely well. Next, I noticed that energy and stamina were increasing.

One day, about two weeks after I began the Zone program, I had been through an extraordinarily busy and challenging day seeing patients, some of whom were quite ill. Finally, it was five o'clock. There was one more new patient to see. That usually meant at least an hour and a half of intense concentration and communication. To do that after a hard day, I usually had to focus my energy and attention hard, and struggle to get through it. That afternoon, I was astonished to realize that my energy and mental clarity were as good as they had been when I started seeing patients that morning! This was even more impressive than the back and elbow pain going away. I did that evaluation with great enjoyment of the ease and energy that I experienced. I also appreciated the mental clarity that enabled me to quickly and easily understand the roots of the patient's serious health problem, communicate with her in a useful way about it, and help her create a workable recovery program. The increased mental clarity and stamina have been a joy to me from that day until this.

The beautiful bonus from the program is I have required an hour less sleep out of every twenty-four. For a physician who is writing a book while carrying a busy daily schedule, this extra hour a day is a precious gift. Soon after I entered the Zone, as Sears puts it, I began to wake up at 4:00 or 4:30 a.m. instead of 5:00 or 5:30. At first, I thought I ought to go back to sleep, but then realized I did not need to go back to sleep. I was rested, refreshed, and eager to get to work on *Healthspan.* I would bet I am not the only person who could use another productive hour in the day.

So this was my gift from the Zone: disappearance of acute and chronic soreness and stiffness, substantially improved energy, stamina, mental clarity, and reduced need for sleep. I soon realized that the Zone is as important to me on the physical level as meditation is on the consciousness level. For twenty-one years, I enhanced the functioning of my Higher Self with meditation. Now, I had an intervention of equal power to anchor the other pole of my Whole Self—the biochemical. With firm anchor points at both poles, productivity, quality of life and mission fulfillment all increased.

Just as when I learned the benefits of meditation twenty-one years ago, when I began to use the Zone program, I eagerly introduced my patients to it. Many of those who began to use it experienced benefits equal to, or greater than, mine. Here are some examples.

A fifty-something teacher had been disabled by severe chemical sensitivities. She was a virtual prisoner in her own house, because even minute exposures to environmental chemicals, such as walking down the detergent aisle in the supermarket or getting a whiff of automobile exhaust on the street, made her deathly ill. Not only that, but she had been depressed for as long as she could remember. After a few weeks in the Zone, her depression had diminished about seventy per cent. In a few more weeks, energy was much better. She was astonished to find that she could now negotiate the detergent aisle without getting sick. By that time, she was having some days completely free of depression. She said, "I feel like I'm from another planet! I never knew how it felt not to be depressed. If I ever want to remember, all I have to do is get out of the Zone. Then the depression is back within hours."

Another woman in her middle years consulted me because of chronic fatigue. In a follow up consultation she said, "After I had been doing the Zone program for about two weeks, I woke up one morning and found that I had enough energy to easily get out of bed. Now I can do brisk twenty to thirty minute walks with no strain. Before the Zone, that felt like trying to climb Mt. Everest. My sleep is much improved. Before the Zone, I used to feel about the same whether I was asleep or awake. I never could get into a sound sleep; then, when I woke up, I couldn't get completely awake. Now, I go into a deep, dead-to-the-world sleep. When I wake up, I'm really awake and alert. My mind is so clear I can see how I used to second guess and sabotage myself with negative thinking."

Another woman in her fifties consulted me because of fatigue and arthritis. Her experience after a few weeks in the Zone was "My joints hurt very little anymore and my energy is better than it's been in a long time. I've been low on energy for so long that I'd forgotten how it felt to have plenty. My digestion is better, too. I wake up earlier and feel rested and refreshed. It's wonderful having another hour in my day!"

A fifty-year-old college professor consulted me because of brain fog and emotional instability so severe that he was afraid he was going crazy. He had been checking his blood sugar and found that it would sometimes go as low as 40 milligrams. I prescribed the Zone. After he had been following the protocol for three or four days he was astonished to find the brain fog gone, the emotional instability completely relieved, and his blood sugar stabilized in the 60's. He reported that his energy and general experience of well being were much improved.

A young attorney consulted me for depression so severe that he had been considering suicide. I prescribed the full Healthspan Center recovery program that included meditation, appropriate physical activity, nutrition that included the Zone, and tyrosine, an antidepressant amino acid. Within six days, he had fully recovered. I had been using the other components of the Healthspan program for years and knew what they were capable of doing. I had expected full recovery in six weeks to six months, not six days. I have to conclude that the addition of the Zone was a major factor in the difference.

The most consistent report that I hear from my patients and friends who are in the Zone is, "When I'm in the Zone I feel peaceful." There are variations on this theme. One woman who entered the Zone after I prescribed it for her schizophrenic son, told me that not only does the pain in her body go away, but her "outlook on life is better". Sometimes I hear that a person becomes so much calmer that things that used to be irritating now hardly cause a ripple.

The most dramatic calming effect is in children who have ADHD. The most rapid and favorable response in children who have this problem has come from a combination of the Zone and neurofeedback, but I have seen spectacularly good results with the Zone program alone.

What is going on here? Part of it is that eicosanoids balance neurotransmitters, which are the final common pathway in determining mood, mind, and behavior. The 30-30-40 balance of macronutrients balances insulin and glucagon. The appropriate balance of insulin and glucagon balances the eicosanoids. The balanced eicosanoids balance neurotransmitters. The results are often wonderful.

By now, you can begin to understand my enthusiasm about the Zone. Let us consider some additional reasons it produces such spectacular results in so many people. You may recall from reading Chapter 2 that excess free radicals are the final common pathway of disease and premature aging. The other critical factor in premature aging is advanced glycosylation end products (AGES). Free radicals are produced when there is an excess of pro-inflammatory eicosanoids. AGES are produced when blood sugar control is poor and blood sugar stays too high for too long. The Zone nutrition program controls both of these problems. This is why it hews to the root of disease and premature aging, those two mortal enemies of the 100-year healthspan.

Sears has clearly presented the details of how and why the Zone works so well and how to do the program. I will not try to re-invent that wheel here. I do strongly encourage you to get a copy of it. You will probably be fascinated to read some brilliant medical detective work, and how you can put it to work right away to enhance the quality of your life within days. As you do so, you will substantially improve your prospects for claiming your natural birthright. *The Zone* has been a number one national bestseller and has sold over one million copies.

Considering the benefits of the program, it is surprising that it is not even more widely known and used. There are several reasons for this. Perhaps the most important is that it represents a paradigm shift away from the conventional nutritional wisdom that the most wholesome diet is high carbohydrate, low fat and low protein. This is the optimum diet for fattening cattle for market, but it is dead wrong for at least seventy-five percent of the human population. Sears clearly explains why, but that does not alter the fact that whenever there is a paradigm shift, there is a lot of conflict and emotional uproar. In fact, the nutritional establishment is outraged against the book. One of my friends, Dr. Rudolph Wiley, has pointed out that whenever there is a paradigm shift, those who had been doing well in the old paradigm will vigorously attack and try to discredit the new one. This is happening.

I have read one conventional nutritionist say that The Zone, "...is a very dangerous diet and should be avoided." The Zone is criticized in the nutritional establishment for being "high protein and high fat." It is neither. In fact, it is adequate protein and moderate fat. It delivers the ratio of macronutrients that human beings evolved over hundreds of thousands of years to thrive on. The nutritional establishment's high carbohydrate, low fat, low protein diet is the disease diet that humans have suffered under for the last five thousand years. The disease diet began with the development of standing agriculture and abundant, dense carbohydrates in the form of grains and grain products. Paleoanthropologists used to wonder why signs of degenerative disease first appeared in human skeletons about five thousand years ago. Once they read *The Zone*, they need wonder no longer. Sears' gift to humankind is the power to return to the level of vigor, health, and physiologic efficiency that our remote ancestors enjoyed throughout most of human history, but not for the last five thousand years. In spite of all this, the nutritional establishment is raging and railing against the Zone, and people who are impressed by the establishment may be afraid to try it.

Another thing slowing acceptance of the Zone program is that it calls for a change in the way we look at food. Instead of being viewed as a recreational, reward, and comfort substance, the Zone requires us to view food primarily as a powerful drug that is to be taken, like any powerful drug, at specified times and in carefully controlled amounts. For those who live to eat, this does not sound like an attractive proposition. Yet, Zone nutrition is inherently delicious and fun. While the basic approach is that food is a powerful drug to be taken in precise doses, Zone—favorable foods can be exquisitely delicious and widely varied. In addition to the enjoyment of eating good food, there is the intellectual satisfaction of arranging to eat it in the proportions that balance your biochemistry.

Most people in this country can find delicious food, but only those in the Zone have the double pleasure of enjoying the food and getting the delightful results from eating it in the proper ratios. Ultimately, there is no food that tastes as good as being healthy feels. Fortunately, with the Zone you get both. Those who eat to live as joyfully, healthily, and productively as possible will love it. Even those who live to eat will find, if they will try the program for a few weeks, that their enjoyment of food increases, to say nothing of their enjoyment of other aspects of their lives. How can you eat less and enjoy it more? Try the Zone for a couple of weeks; find out!

Another factor that keeps some people out of the Zone is a strange thing about hidden or delayed food allergy. Some food allergic reactions happen within minutes. Others may wait up to four days to show up. With those delayed allergies, most people do not make the connection between the food and the symptom. With delayed food allergies, we can get addicted to foods that we are allergic to! This happens because, when there is a delayed food allergy, the body will often turn part of the food into a substance called exorphin. This strange molecule goes and sits on the same binding sites on brain cells that narcotics sit on, with similarly powerful effects on mood, mind, and behavior. Many people are addicted to carbohydrates. Carbohydrate craving can be a powerful addiction, sometimes nearly uncontrollable. Just as a heroin addict has a hard time going cold turkey, so a carbo-hydrate addict (I know, I have been one) can have a hard time doing the carbohydrate reduction called for by the Zone. I have heard that addicts who have suddenly stopped using both heroin and sugar, say that sugar withdrawal is worse. No one has to go cold turkey off carbohydrates to do the Zone, but there may be a substantial decrease in the quantity eaten in order to achieve the 40-30-30 balance. Fortunately, the withdrawal reaction lasts only four or five days, but while it is going on, it can be intense.

Perhaps the greatest obstacle for many people who are con-sidering doing the Zone program is that they just do not believe how much better they will feel and function in the Zone. I would not believe it if I had not experienced it. I certainly did not expect it. As more and more people experience these benefits and talk about them with others, the disbelief factor will diminish, but it is still something you have to experience to believe.

I leave this section with the enthusiastic recommendation that the next book you read after you finish this one be *The Zone*.

Dealing with the toxic food problem

Earlier in this chapter, you read a discussion of the impor-tance of pure water. Non-toxic food is just as important. Trying to balance biochemistry with poisoned food is like trying to smother a fire with gasoline. Unfortunately, nontoxic food is even harder to get than pure water. If the EPA can be believed, all of the food that comes from the supermarket is poisoned to one degree or another—unless it comes from the organic section in the supermarket.

There has been enough discussion of the poisoning of the standard American diet in the chapter on Dream Destroyers. Now it is time to talk about how to solve the problem. The first step is to eat organically grown food whenever possible. More supermarkets are offering organic food. If yours is not, I encour-age you to talk to the produce manager. Health food stores can often refer you to an organic farmer or may sell organic food.

The second step is to eat the less heavily poisoned foods. Meat is by far the worst offender, because animals bioaccumulate poisons. When you eat grain, you just get the poison that was on that grain. When you eat meat you get the poison that was on the grain that the animal ate, which was a lot more than you are likely to eat, particularly if you are in the Zone. Whenever possible, get your daily Zone prescription of protein from organically raised meat, tofu, or protein powders, particularly rice, whey or soy. There are now several soy-based, processed foods that are palatable, tasting something like hamburger and sausage.

The third part of your strategy is to take plenty of the nutrients your body must have to detoxify itself. More about that later.

The fourth and elegant step in the strategy is to become an organic gardener. This is such an important and delightful way to the 100-year healthspan that we will probably write a book about it as part of the *Healthspan* series. Here is a preview. Gardening is one of the few activities that simultaneously balances biochemistry, energy and consciousness. The title of the textbook for biointensive gardening, which we do, is *How To Grow More Vegetables Than You Ever Thought Possible On Less Land Than You Can Imagine.* The author is John Jeavons. The title tells the truth. Even if you live twenty stories up in a high rise, you can still garden in a window box and get Healthspan mileage out of it. In the average-size backyard, you can probably grow enough vegetables to feed a family of two for a year. Even if you do not want to take up yard space growing wholesome food, you might consider the European method. Europeans, being generally more civilized than Americans, interplant vegetables with ornamental shrubs and flowers around their houses. This can be pleasing to the eye as well as to the palette. Stay tuned for a title that may be *Cultivating Your 100-Year Healthspan In Your Garden.*

Let us now consider nutritional supplementation.

NUTRITIONAL SUPPLEMENTATION

Why take nutritional supplements? After all, for years the position of the American Dietetic Association and the medical establishment has been, "Eat a balanced diet and you don't need nutritional supplements. You get everything you need in the balanced diet."

There are several fallacies in this quaint, archaic notion. First, less than 10% of the U.S. population eats what the nutritional establishment would consider a "balanced diet." That is probably fortunate because the nutritional establishment has the balance all wrong. The U.S.D.A.'s food pyramid is grossly excessive in carbohydrate. By now, you know something about the havoc that creates in the body-mind. Since the "balanced diet" is not balanced, and hardly anybody eats it anyway, it obviously cannot deliver the vitamins, minerals, essential fatty acids and accessory nutrients that are required for reasonable health, let alone the 100-year healthspan. That is the first part of the answer.

The second part is that, after reading Dream Destroyers and Birthright Burglars, you know what a number has been done on your food before you buy it from the supermarket. You probably recall that it has been grown on mineral-depleted land, hybridized for appearance at the expense of nutritional content, poisoned, and "partitioned." It is thus in pathetic condition to deliver the nutrients that you need.

The third part of the answer is that, since we live in an egregiously polluted environment, so that we poison ourselves every time we eat, drink, and breathe, we must be able to detoxify efficiently. Your body's detoxification system depends on vitamins, minerals, amino acids, and essential fatty acids. It needs these nutrients and it needs lots of them. Even if you did Zone nutrition with organically grown food, which is the best nutritional combination we know, you would still need substantial nutritional supplementation in order to have optimum detoxification power. These are the reasons that we consider nutritional supplementation essential to the attainment of the 100-year healthspan.

Next question: what and how much? You may be surprised at how few things this physician, trained in nutritional medicine, is going to recommend. Please understand that these recommendations are for people who are in good health and want to stay that way. For people who are sick, there is a vast array of nutritional interventions that may be remarkably useful. In subsequent books, we plan to make suggestions for specific programs for nutritional supplementation that are likely to be useful in treating particular conditions. If you are not in good health, do not wait. Read *Dr. Wright's Guide to Healing with Nutrition* and subscribe to his *Nutrition and Healing* newsletter. There are many other good books and newsletters on balancing biochemistry. In addition to *Nutrition and Healing,* we subscribe to and recommend to our patients, *Health & Healing* by Julian Whitaker, M.D., *Self Healing* by Andrew Weil, M.D., and *Health Wisdom for Women* by Christiane Northrup, M.D. Each of these publications has its unique approach and value. You will benefit from reading them all. The more serious your health problems, the more of them you should read-and heed.

In this book, we are dealing with the core program for healthy people. For those who are not healthy, the core program is even more important. Using it will increase the probability of recovery from disease, but it needs to be enhanced with specific nutrients beneficial in the particular condition.

The foundation

Here is the core program for nutritional supplementation. The foundation for the program is a high potency, broad- spectrum multiple vitamin and mineral supplement. The one that I have found works best for most people is Basic Preventive 3 or 5, by Advanced Medical Nutrition, Inc. (AMNI). Why 3 or 5? Basic Preventive-3 contains iron. Women who have menstrual periods and anyone who has iron deficiency should take this one. Everybody else should take Basic Preventive-5, which has no iron. Iron, like everything else, needs to be in the appropriate balance in the body. Too little makes you anemic and weak. Too much causes excessive free radical activity. By now, you know what that means. The Basic Preventive formulas are available in tablets or capsules. Use the capsules. These are preferable because they may improve absorption and they eliminate the risk of allergic reactions to excipients. Excipients are everything in the tablet that is not active ingredient: flavoring, coloring, binders, fillers, and lubricants. If you think you may be allergic to gelatin used to make the capsules, simply open them and dump the contents into food or liquid. It will not taste good, but it will taste better than an allergic reaction feels.

Recent research has established the need for more vitamins D and E than we thought were optimum. We now know that vitamin D functions as a neurohormone to protect against seasonal affective disorder and as an immune system inhancer, as well as aiding calcium absorption. Vitamin E, in higher doses, is an important protector of nerve cells. It must be in the form of mixed tocopherols for best results.

The Basic Preventive formula has not yet caught up with this new knowledge. For best results, in addition to Basic Preventive, take vitamin D (available from Bronson Pharmaceutical) 400 IU twice daily, and vitamin E plus mixed tocopherols (AMNI) 400 IU once daily. Phone numbers for ordering are in Resources.

Vitamin C

The next supplement is vitamin C, chemically known as ascorbic acid. It is nature's premier detoxifier, and one of the best free radical scavengers. There are two options for taking vitamin C for the 100-year healthspan. One is to take the maximum amount possible without activating enzymes that use vitamin C at an accelerated rate. This happens to be 6 grams of ascorbic acid per day. If you are taking ascorbic acid, you need to dose four times a day, because it is fast in and fast out. The optimum schedule would be 1.5 grams with each meal and at bedtime. If you do not want to dose that often, you can use Ester-C, 2 grams, twice daily. It gives better tissue levels and stays in the tissues longer than ascorbic acid.

Why would anybody want to take ascorbic acid instead of Ester-C? The only reasons I know are that it is much cheaper and you do not have to be concerned about getting too much calcium. Ester-C has about 100mg of calcium in each gram (1000 mg) of ascorbic acid. If you take more than 15 grams of Ester-C daily, or take smaller amounts together with other calcium-containing supplements, you may exceed 1500 mg of calcium daily. You should do that only under the supervision of a knowledgeable healthcare professional. If you are wondering why on earth anyone would be taking more than 15 grams of Ester-C daily, read on.

The other way of using vitamin C is to take as much each day as your body will absorb. We learned about this from Robert Cathcart, M.D., a leading authority on high-dose vitamin C. We call his method the Ascorbate Protocol. (Ascorbate is a shorter name for Vitamin C.) Your body-mind is astonishingly intelligent: it knows exactly how much vitamin C it needs at any given time in order to detoxify itself and deal with any infection or allergic reaction that is going on. It will absorb what it needs and eliminate the rest through loose or watery bowel movements. In the appendix we have a protocol that tells you how to ask your body how much vitamin C it needs on any given day to feel and function its best. Study the protocol and you will know how to ask the question and listen for the answer. Once you can do that, you have taken a significant step towards your 100-year healthspan.

Vitamin C is a threshold substance. That means that below the threshold of your bowel tolerance (the amount you can take with digestive system comfort), nothing much happens. Reach the threshold, however, and wow, something sure happens! What will probably happen is that your energy increases along with your mental clarity, minor aches and pains go away, and major ones get better. If you are having allergic reactions, such as hay fever or sinus congestion, they are likely to improve from 50 to 90%. These benefits are maintained as long as you maintain your bowel tolerance level. This can be a little tricky at first because your vitamin C requirement will vary from day to day depending on how much stress you are under and whether your body-mind is dealing with an infection, allergic reaction, or trauma. For example, when I am healthy, my gut tolerance is about 30 grams (30,00 milligrams per day). If I get a severe infection, which has not happened in years, I may take up to 99 grams in twenty-four hours before I exceed my gut tolerance and kick the infection out.

William Blake, a wonderfully wise and aware poet and philosopher, wrote, "You never know what is enough until you know what is more than enough." That is how it is with the Ascorbate Protocol. You take enough to get a couple of watery bowel movements, then back off slightly until you are taking the maximum amount possible with complete digestive comfort. Remember that it is going to vary from day to day. Do not worry about that; soon you will get so good at reading the subtle messages from your body-mind that you know how much to take at any given time in order to get maximum benefit without offending your gut. Used in this way, Vitamin C will substantially enhance of your probability of the 100-year healthspan and improve your comfort and safety every day.

With so many benefits coming from the gut tolerance protocol for vitamin C, why would anybody want to take less? One reason is that there is some persistent misinformation circulating about vitamin C. Probably the scariest thing is the allegation that it causes kidney stones. This was disproved years ago but it persists as a medical myth. It is true that if you take big doses of vitamin C you have to take adequate amounts of magnesium and B6 to protect against kidney stones. There are adequate amounts of B6 and magnesium in either of the Basic Preventive formulas. If you have had kidney stones, you should take large doses of C under the supervision of a knowledgeable nutritional health professional, preferably one that can order laboratory tests to see if you are excreting excessive amounts of oxalate, from which kidney stones may be made. If you have never had kidney stones and if you are taking Basic Preventive or any similar formula, I do not think you need be concerned about the medical myth.

The only real reason I know for not doing the gut tolerance protocol is that you may induce enzymes that use vitamin C rapidly. If you suddenly stop taking vitamin C after these enzymes have been activated, they may continue to use it so rapidly that, with no new vitamin C coming in, your tissue levels can go too low. This can result in a condition called "rebound scurvy" —not a good thing to have. When you have scurvy, rebound or otherwise, your immune function drops precipitously, you bleed excessively, old wounds may break open, and you are susceptible to shock, exhaustion, and depression. This is bad enough under the best circumstances; but suppose, God forbid, you are in an automobile accident and the EMT people pick you up unconscious out of your vehicle. If you are doing the gut tolerance protocol, they need to know to give you intravenous vitamin C until you can take it again by mouth, and they had better do it. Otherwise, you and they may get into deep trouble, because if you are critically injured you surely do not want rebound scurvy. On the other hand, if they give you enough intravenous ascorbate, your chances of recovery are much better than they would be if you had not been taking vitamin C in the first place. Our orthopedic surgeon friend gave his patients vitamin C 100 grams (100,000 milligrams) intravenously during the first 24 hours after surgery. Not one of those patients ever had a wound infection.

If you decide to do the protocol for more than two weeks at a time, always wear a medic alert necklace or bracelet that says "See wallet card." See the protocol in the appendix for the information to put on the wallet card. This does not guarantee that emergency medical personnel will give you the vitamin C after they read the card. There is still a substantial portion of the

medical establishment that thinks that vitamins do not do anything, so there is no reason to use them. They may also think that
the amount of vitamin C you are taking is a lethal dose. Even
with the medical alert system, you still may not get the vitamin
C. If you do the Protocol, be sure that those close to you, who
would be making decisions about your care if you were unconscious, know to insist on your getting vitamin C. In a severe situation, they might even need to mention to an attending
physician who is refusing to give you adequate doses of Vitamin
C, that your attorney is seriously concerned about the harm that
may come to you as a result.

With all these hazards and hassles, why would anyone want
to do the Ascorbate Protocol? Many people feel and function so
much better on the protocol that they are willing to run the risk. It
is like saying, with all the risks and hazards out there on the highway, why would anybody ever leave home? It comes down to the
risk-benefit ratio and how you balance those two things out.

One way of deciding this is to do the Protocol for two weeks.
You will not induce the enzymes in two weeks, but you will discover how much benefit you get. If you then think the
risk-benefit ratio is favorable, keep on doing it. If you do not
think so, then drop back to six grams of ascorbic acid or four
grams of Ester-C per day and forget about rebound scurvy.

If you choose the latter program, you can still use the gut tolerance protocol if you start to get sick. If you use it that way, the
main risk is that you will not be aggressive enough to stop the infection before it gets a grip on you. When I first read Cathcart's
publications on the ascorbate protocol and intravenous vitamin
C, I was so impressed that Genevieve and I flew to California to
spend an evening with him, learning how to use these treatments. During that visit, he told us that you know within twenty
minutes whether or not you have taken an adequate dose. If you
are getting sick, have taken a dose of vitamin C, and you are not
starting to feel better or get diarrhea within twenty minutes, that
means you did not take enough. You should then take the next

dose, making it larger, as directed in the protocol. The protocol says dose every hour; that is conservative. If you are in a hurry to feel better, do as Cathcart said. It took me years to get aggressive enough for maximum benefit. I still do not take enough fast enough sometimes.

That is the vitamin C story. It is important enough to justify the space it has taken.

Other important supplements

There are two other supplements that belong in the core program for the 100-year healthspan: calcium and flax seed meal. I recommend calcium in an absorbable form such as citrate (calcium citrate) 500 milligrams, twice daily. If you are taking Ester-C, adjust the calcium citrate dose so that you do not get more the 1500 mg of calcium from supplements daily. I am assuming that you do not use large amounts of dairy products. I consider them health hazards for all except blood type B's. If you have had kidney stones, you still need to be under medical supervision and have the oxalate test run. Sometimes that much calcium will increase calcium excretion and the risk of more stone formation. If you have never had kidney stones, just go ahead and take your calcium. Do not use calcium carbonate, as in Tums. It is the most poorly absorbed form, particularly in folks over fifty. It is likely to make the stomach so alkaline that digestion and all mineral absorption is impaired, and the risk of yeast overgrowth is increased. Tums are fine as an antacid, certainly better than any of the aluminum-containing products, but not satisfactory for calcium supplementation.

The fourth supplement is flaxseed meal. I recommend it because it is rich in omega three essential fatty acid, which is desperately scarce in the standard American diet. The omega threes are essential to control of free radical activity. In addition, the flax meal normalizes cholesterol, protects against constipation and colon cancer, and helps with weight loss by absorbing so much water that you feel full without eating so much. You have to mill your flaxseed into meal just before you eat it because it gets rancid quickly. The seeds mill as easily as coffee beans in a coffee mill. See the Resources section for a source.

If milling flaxseed is too much trouble, take a tablespoonful of flaxseed oil each day. It makes a good salad oil or dressing on hot veggies or bread. Do not try to cook with it: heat makes it break down into toxic substances. With the oil, you get the omega threes, but not the other benefits of flax meal.

Once you attain the halfway point in your 100-year healthspan, we recommend that you begin to take ginkgo biloba. Ginkgo-D, by MMS Pro, is a reliable brand. The dose is 60 mg twice daily. Ginkgo improves blood flow throughout the body, particularly in the brain. It is a powerful antioxidant, protecting the brain. Many studies have demonstrated its ability to protect and improve brain function.

With those four or five supplements, you have your core 100-year healthspan program. There are dozens of other supplements you could take and some you should take if you have health problems, but if you are healthy and want to stay that way until you are 100, we suggest that you keep your supplement program simple and commit more of your resources higher up in your Whole Self. As you penetrate deeper into your 100-year healthspan, there are some other things you need to take. This is such a big and important issue that we are addressing it, as well as many others, in our next book, *The 100-Year Healthspan for Folks Over Fifty*.

HORMONES

There are two hormones that you might want to consider as part of your 100-year healthspan program: melatonin and DHEA. I do not recommend either of these for routine use for people under fifty, although melatonin can be useful at any age for reducing jetlag.

Before going into detail about hormones, it is time to restate a basic Birthright principle. Balance at all levels of life ultimately comes from balanced consciousness. When consciousness is balanced, as described in Chapter 4, there is automatic balancing of energy and biochemistry. The more you do at the level of balancing consciousness, or awareness, the less you have to do on the biochemical level. That is a fundamental principle and that is where I recommend you put the majority of your attention. However, all that takes some time to work out; in the meantime, you may want to have the benefit of some hormones. It is important to get benefit and not side effects.

For people over fifty and melatonin doses of 3 milligrams or less, taken an hour before bedtime, there is no indication of serious short-term side effects. Some people get depressed, some have daytime drowsiness or feel spacey, but these problems usually go away promptly upon stopping melatonin. It has not been used long enough for us to know what the long-term problems may be; but, so far, so good. Most people who take it believe they get improved quality of sleep. Bottom line: if you want to take melatonin to improve the quality of sleep and you are over fifty, start with one milligram at bedtime. Adjust the dose up to a maximum of 3 milligrams and down to a minimum of one-tenth a milligram to find what works best for you.

The other hormone is DHEA. It has been hailed as the fountain of youth. As mentioned earlier, this is a naive view of the complexity of life; but for some people over fifty, DHEA has improved energy, strength, and mood. The cancer risk connection is not clear. There is some indication it reduces cancer risk, but recent reports suggest that long-term use may increase risk of prostate and breast cancer. DHEA is a powerful adrenal hormone. It is capable of producing serious side effects. It seems remarkable that the FDA has not tried to regulate DHEA, while it has vigorously suppressed innocuous substances such as flax oil, evening primrose oil and saw palmetto extract.

The most important thing about using DHEA is to test to see if you need it. If you need it, it can help you. If you do not need it and you take it anyway, it can hurt you. It can suppress production of another important adrenal hormone, cortisol. It may also increase the risk of breast and prostate cancer. There are several ways of testing, all of which are available to physicians. For a screening test, I prefer to use saliva which tells me what is coming out of cells rather than what is in blood waiting to go in. The salivary test is available from at least two laboratories. Contact information is in the Resources section of the Appendix. If testing indicates low levels of DHEA, then supplementation is indicated and should be done under the guidance of a health care provider who is knowledgeable about using the hormone and able to order and interpret the tests.

Too little DHEA is safer than too much. I usually start with 5 milligrams daily for women and 10 milligrams daily for men, gradually increasing the dose to 15 milligrams and 30 milligrams respectively. Then we retest. The retest will be done on urine. The reason is that there are two important downstream metabolites of DHEA, epiandosterone, and eticholanolone.

Sometimes, due to a quirk of adrenal biochemistry, these two downstream hormones will be elevated, although DHEA is normal, or low. When this happens, low DHEA is probably an automatic adjustment by the body-mind to protect against excessive levels of the two downstream hormones. We do not know what excessive levels of these will do over a long period, but there may be a connection with the increased incidence of prostate and breast cancer. Too many people had their health devastated in the cortisone disaster that followed the discovery of that substance in the fifties and the use of larger amounts than the body could manage. Let us take warning from their misfortune and not repeat the mistake with DHEA.

DHEA sold in health food stores may or may not be active. I have taken some over the counter DHEA that laboratory testing showed was inert. Pharmaceutical grade DHEA, compounded by a pharmacist, is more reliable. It can be taken by mouth or applied transdermally. A compounding pharmacist in your community can tell you which physicians are prescribing DHEA. For the toll-free number of a national referral service for compounding pharmacists, see the Resources section of the Appendix.

If you do take DHEA, it is best done for a period of six to nine months. During that time, you can act to support your adrenal function, so that you can then wean off DHEA and make a sufficient amount in your own adrenals. The most powerful adrenal supportive practice I know is to spend a half-hour or more twice a day in the mind state of quiet alertness. This has been shown in laboratory studies to significantly increase DHEA output. In men the increase is around 15%, in women around 25%. Every intervention you have read about and will read about in this chapter supports adrenal function by providing adequate quantities of nutrients that the adrenals have to have to function optimally and by reducing your stress load. Since adrenals are the primary shock organ for dealing with overstress, they really appreciate that and will reward you by putting out more of their hormones when needed.

Hormone replacement therapy for women is worth considering, but is beyond the scope of this book, requiring considerable expertise for maximum benefit and minimum side effects. It is important to be aware that the replacement should be done with natural hormones, particularly natural progesterone, and not the synthetic progestins such as Provera, which for many women is an assault on their physiology. There is a growing appreciation for the benefits of natural hormones among gynecologists and you probably would not have to look very long to find one who is knowledgeable in their use.

HERBS

Herbal therapy has a long and distinguished history in dealing with suffering and disease and promoting health. My understanding of the basis of herbal therapy comes from my ayurvedic training. It goes like this: each organ of the body has its own unique vibrational frequency when it is healthy. When, due to stress or trauma, the vibrational frequency changes, there is likely to be disease. It is like a guitar going out of tune when dropped on the floor. The restoration of health requires retuning the organ to its original, healthy frequency.

Each plant has its own vibrational frequency. Some plants possess the same vibrational frequencies of each organ of the body. When an organ has de-tuned, it may be re-tuned by exposure to the vibrations of the appropriate plant or herb. Centuries of experience have shown which herbs are beneficial to which organs. The re-tuning process may be similar to the sympathetic vibration that is set up on the string of a musical instrument when a vibrating tuning fork of the same frequency is held nearby.

Like hormonal therapy, herbal therapy for treatment of illness should be administered by a knowledgeable professional. There are some ayurvedic herbal formulas that I believe are generally useful in fine tuning the energy body and promoting the 100-year healthspan. The premiere formula is called Biochavan. It consists of several herbs which, over thousands of years, have proven their value in promoting health and protecting against disease. This formula is available as a paste that tastes like grape jam. For those who do not like grape jam, the formula is available in tablets. The paste is known as Biochavan 1, the tablets as Biochavan 2. These are available from The Chopra Center for Wellness. Telephone number is in Resources.

The other ayurvedic formulas that I recommend for general use are called Optiman and Optiwoman. These formulas contain herbs that are believed to support and balance the male and female physiologies.

The take away from this section is that the more you do on the level of balancing consciousness, mind, and energy, the less you will need to do to balance biochemistry, because that will largely be taken care of automatically. However, you will still need to do some direct biochemical balancing. In the meantime, while you are learning to work effectively on these higher levels, the direct biochemical balancing procedures can be of great benefit.

Part III
Wisdom for Applying Your Knowledge

Chapter 13

BALANCING WHOLE SELF: STRATEGY

INTRODUCTION

Having read this far, you know that we believe the 100-year healthspan is a possible dream. You probably think so, too, or you would not still be reading. You also know what we believe are the most dangerous hazards to living this dream. More importantly, you understand something about the interventions we consider most likely to empower you to transcend the hazards and enjoy your birthright. Now comes the most valuable, challenging, and exciting part of this experience: putting what you have learned into action. It is time to create your personal, individualized 100-year healthspan program, which will unleash and focus the power of all this knowledge to attain your birthright. You do not have to wait until you are 100 years old to start enjoying your birthright. The enjoyment starts when you begin taking action to claim your birthright. Then the enjoyment grows stronger as you do the program longer. In this chapter, you will find an excellent example in some excerpts from the diary of a woman who has spent several years using some of these interventions to claim her birthright.

In this chapter, we will tell you four strategic principles that you can use in creating your 100-year healthspan program. In the next, we will discuss the tactics for putting your program into action in your daily life. It is only when you carry this knowledge into action that you feel the power, enjoy the exhilaration, and savor the adventure that is potential in this knowledge

FROM BETTY'S JOURNAL

"Saturday, December 17

"How do I feel? Lots of thoughts on my mind. I listened to the first half of Dr. Woodard's tape on the way down and I'm anxious to hear the rest. It was so exciting to hear and it rang so true. I wanted to clap and cheer. I really feel that as the next couple of years go by I will look and feel so much better. It's so exciting to think about it. I'm really going to get better and better. Over the last year, I've gone from feeling absolutely horrible to feeling really good most of the time. Now I know that over the next year I'm going to go from good to fabulous. I am going to beat the yeast—I am. And I'm going to become flexible and mobile and feel so good. And be able to dance and move; that's going to be wonderful. And I honestly feel that that's more important than looks. My looks will improve too, and that's going to make me so happy, but that will be a side effect of the primary thing going on. My looks will improve as a result of my returning health, but my health is my motivation, not my looks. This is a big change of attitude for me.

"Gosh, when I think back to when I turned 40, and how I felt that year—'93—I was so depressed, so depressed, because I felt that my life was over, that I'd never look good and feel good again. Deep down, I felt that my immune system was dysfunctioning so severely that I would get cancer within the next 10 years and die a horrible death. Now I feel that—give me a couple of years—and my immune system is going to get so great, that even if I did get cancer, I'd beat it.

"The timing of Dr. Woodard's workshop is so perfect, because now I really believe and understand what he's saying with my intellect and my feelings. A year ago, I would have heard it with my intellect only and it wouldn't have been half as effective. Like so much of what's going on with Dr. Woodard, it's coming at the right time, when I'm ready. Yes, I am going to have a hundred-year healthspan and I'm finally so happy to be over 40. Because it doesn't mean getting old and sick and ugly. It means getting wise and knowledgeable and glowingly healthy. It feels so wonderful to know that getting older means getting better. Not the way it's usually meant—not like wine. But meaning getting healthier and physically better. And I know from the experience of the last year, that you can't truly be happy when you're physically ill. Nowadays I feel so happy that I feel exhilarated. A lot of that comes from all the blessings I've had for years— my husband, my kids, my home, my job. But so much of it comes from the sheer overwhelming joy of feeling so good!"

This patient has done as she said she would. In the three years since she made the above entry in her journal, she has steadily used and evolved the program you have been reading about. At the time of this journal entry, she was working mainly on the physical level of her Whole Self. Over the next three years, she began to develop the mental and spiritual levels concurrently. One by one, her symptoms and diseases have fallen away. She recently told me that she has been delighted to be able to ride bicycles with her husband and children again. This was the first time in many years, and it was during the heaviest pollen season in years.

Before she began her *Healthspan* program, even brief exposure outdoors to this pollen would have left her wheezing and aching so severely that bicycle riding would have been out of the question. In addition to recovering her health and ability to function and enjoy life, she has dealt with three major crises in her family. They have not been fun, but she managed her responsibilities in them and has contributed to favorable outcomes, without getting sick again. She is essentially on her own now, calling occasionally to let us know about her progress and to ask about how to address some particular issue. Here is a recent journal entry in which she summarizes her experience of the three years since the first one.

"Monday, May 12, 1997

"How do I feel? It's been almost 4 years since I started seeing Dr. Woodard. How have things changed? Well, the change is so dramatic that I think back and remember how I used to be, and I wonder how I made it through that time. I remember getting out of bed in the morning and wondering how I would make it though the day. Sometimes I would be crying from sheer exhaustion and I could hardly get my makeup on. Then, all through the day I would count the hours left and pray to get through them. On the days I didn't work, I just laid on the couch day and night, exhausted and sick. What a life! .

"Then I found Dr. Woodard and began the healing process, which is still going on. This healing process has been just that—a process—and I've learned so much. Many times, I've had to remind myself of what Dr. Woodard told me when he said I would take two steps forward and one step back. That's sure what happened! For the longest time I thought that if we could just find the right medication, or figure out the one thing I was allergic to, then I'd get well—just like magic—take a pill, be well. Of course that's not the way it was, but it's the way I wanted it to be. I'd get so frustrated and furious when I took those inevitable steps back. And then, I'd get so depressed. Sometimes the only thing that gave me hope was that Dr. Woodard would tell me he was sure I'd get better and he was certain. So, even though I had doubts and I was scared, I'd focus on his certainty and hang in there.

"It took me a long time to realize that health is a state of balance—a balance of so many things and that when one part of the body gets knocked out of balance it affects all the rest of the body too. So now, I strive to keep things balanced. It's really that simple. And if I get to feeling lousy, I realize that it'll pass—it's just temporary—not a lifelong condition. What a wonderful feeling it is to know that!

"So now, almost four years later, I look back and can hardly believe how lousy I used to feel every day. I feel a sense of well being almost every single day now, usually all day long. In addition, that feeling is euphoric. About halfway through, I'd get an occasional glimpse of that great feeling, but now it's just about a constant presence. Which is just amazing to me. It's so wonderful to have the energy to function well every day and also to have the mental state to enjoy every day.

"I find that I withstand every day stresses very well, and even extraordinary stresses too. I'd had some painful life changes in the last year or so, and I find that I came through them OK. Being healthy just seems to give me so much more latitude physically and emotionally. I can handle so much more and still be calm and happy. It just amazes me.

"I still have a long way to go. I need to lose weight, there's more fine-tuning to be done with my body and we're working on that. I have so much more to learn and I love that! What I've learned so far has been so invaluable and exciting that I love the thought that there's a lot more to learn. In addition, I'm not talking about learning about medical data, physiology, although I've learned a lot about that too. But what I've learned about life, other human beings, and myself has been invaluable and wonderful. So now I'm cherishing this process of healing, the same process that used to make me so mad in the beginning. I'm thankful every day that I feel so good. I'm deeply grateful for the chance to be healthier and live and love the people around me. Every day is a gift. I even hope to be here long enough to learn to love everyone around me, to be able to reach that elusive goal of being able to banish anger and bitterness and hate completely. I keep trying! See how far I've come! I no longer pray for the strength to crawl through the day; now I find joy in every single day."

We are grateful to Betty for letting us use her words to describe her experiences with using the Healthspan principles. She communicates in a way we never could, not only the facts but also the feelings, joys, and frustrations of the process. The *spirit* of the process of claiming her birthright shines through in these journal entries.

Yes, there are frustrations as well as joys in this process of claiming your birthright, but the frustrations neither dim the spirit nor outweigh the joy.

A friend used to say, "Think how happy you would be if you lost everything you had—and then got it back again." This is powerfully true where health is concerned. Some of the happiest people we ever see are those who have lost their health and are getting it back again. Being associated with the process that brings such happiness is one of the rewards of doing our work and fulfilling our missions.

As delicious as this happiness of recovery is, there is an even deeper, longer, stronger happiness associated with nurturing health to higher and higher levels. This kind of happiness comes *after* recovery from disease and injury. It releases energy and power that you can use however you choose. If you choose to use them to fulfill your mission, you compound the happiness and the power. This process strongly supports attainment of the 100-year healthspan.

Betty's experience reminds us of a fundamental difference between conventional and holistic medicine. The difference is in the attitudes toward becoming long living, an achievement that conventional medicine calls aging. Remember what you read in Chapter 2 about Abkhasia, the "longevity belt," where there are no old people but there are plenty of long living people? The position of conventional medicine is that aging is an incurable, universally fatal disease which must be held at bay as long as possible. The position of holistic medicine is that as we live longer, we get wiser. We can use this wisdom to make choices that continue to improve functioning, fulfillment, and quality of life until we are ready to "drop the body" as Carl's granddad did in the episode described in the Epilogue.

Now comes the opportunity to discover ways to apply this wisdom so that you can improve *your* functioning and strengthen your experience of happiness and fulfillment. That is part of your birthright. Learn! Act! Enjoy!

STRATEGIC *Principle 1*

A competent self-healing mechanism is essential to achieving the 100-year healthspan.

Deep within every cell of your body, at the level of DNA, there is a self-healing mechanism that is operating at every moment. When fully activated, this mechanism has awesome power. More than forty years of experience in medical practice has led me to believe that it has the potential to heal any disease or injury. The sufficient activation of this self-healing mechanism is essential to the 100-year healthspan because, as you know from reading the chapter on Dream Destroyers and Birthright Burglars, and from your own experiences of living in the world, it is a jungle out there—and there are tigers in it. If you walk long enough in a jungle with tigers, you are going to get clawed. A hundred years is a long walk indeed, so you will get clawed from time to time. This means you need to be able to heal quickly and completely. That is what activation of your self-healing mechanism empowers you to do.

STRATEGIC *Principle 2*

The self-healing mechanism is activated by achieving balance and harmony within your Whole Self.

Balance and harmony within your Whole Self means giving to each of the seven levels of your Whole Self the appropriate quality and quantity of attention. The *quality* of attention refers to what *kind* of attention you give to a particular level. For example, quiet alertness is an appropriate kind of attention to give to the level of Pure Consciousness. Partial attention, such as attention divided between Pure Consciousness and watching TV, is not an appropriate quality of attention. The *quantity* of attention refers to *how much* attention you give to a particular level of your Whole Self. For example, a half-hour of exercise daily is, for

some people, an appropriate amount of attention to give to the
energy level of the Whole Self; a half-minute of exercise is not. In
this section, I will tell you what I consider some of the most appropriate kinds of attention to give to each level of your Whole
Self. I will then tell you how you can determine what is the appropriate amount of attention to give to each level.

The appropriate quality of attention: The Healthspan System for Balance and Harmony

The interventions that I am about to suggest to you are the
best of the best of the many I have learned and used in over forty
years of medical practice. It is a joy to bring them to you because
they have worked so well for so many people. I have watched
many patients use them to regain health, happiness, and zest for
life. I have the expectation that, if you use them, they will work
well for you also. The six components of the Healthspan System
are the practice of quiet alertness, the Flick Protocol, appropriate physical activity, appropriate nutrition, fulfillment of life
mission, and mutually satisfying relationships.

These six interventions create balance and harmony on all
seven levels of your Whole Self. Some of them, obviously, work
on more than one level. The practice of quiet alertness, for example, works directly on the levels of Pure Consciousness, Causal
Consciousness, Intellect, and Energy. Since the Whole Self is a
system, quiet alertness has an indirect effect on the remaining
three levels as well. This is one reason that I consider it the most
important part of the Healthspan System. I will now give a brief
description of each part of this system and tell you where to find
the detailed instructions on how to use each component.

Quiet Alertness, regularly practiced, strengthens the
power of attention, which is, as we have explained in Chapter 4,
power for the 100-year healthspan. Other benefits include balancing every level of the Whole Self; dissipating the toxic effects
of overstress, and giving you access to the wisdom, serenity,
and bliss of Pure Consciousness. Since it does so much so well, I
suggest that, if you are going to use only one part of the

Healthspan System, you choose Quiet Alertness. Instructions are in Chapter 5.

The Five Rites of Rejuvenation are ancient Tibetan practices that produce more rejuvenation per minute than anything else that we know. They are unique in our experience, but somewhat resemble an integration of yoga and calisthenics. If you like time-efficiency for increasing energy and comfort in your body-mind, you will love the Five Rites of Rejuvenation. Instructions are in Chapter 12.

Clearing for the Family Tree is a unique system for using skillfully worded prayer and behavioral techniques to neutralize patterns of toxic energy that are passed down in families from generation to generation, contributing to recurring mental and physical disorders. Developed by Denny Ray Johnson, a deeply spiritual naturopath, they offer a way to access an important dimension of healing that is otherwise virtually inaccessible and usually neglected. Instructions are in the Appendix.

Physical Activity—The principle here is "use it or lose it." Many studies have shown that physically active people are healthier longer than sedentary ones. A good example is the Honolulu Study, a large scale, prospective study published in the prestigious *New England Journal of Medicine,* in which 707 men aged 61 through 81 were followed for 12 years. During that time, 208 died. The mortality rate for those who walked more than 2 miles a day was one half that of those who walked less than two miles daily, after mortality rate was adjusted for age. In another study, published in the same journal, physically active, non-smoking men who maintained a healthy body composition (were not obese) became disabled seven years later than sedentary, obese smokers did. When the active men did get disabilities, they recovered faster. Our recommendations for physical activity are in Chapter 11: Balancing Energy.

Appropriate Diet

Let your medicine be your food and your food your medicine.

—Hippocrates

Without proper diet, of medicine there is no use. With proper diet, of medicine there is no need.

—Ayurvedic aphorism

Our recommendations for appropriate diet are in Chapter 13, Balancing Biochemistry.

Healthspan Nutritional Supplements

You may be surprised at how few supplements you need if you do the full Healthspan Program—but the ones I recommend are very important, probably critical.

Recommendations are also in Chapter 13.

Relationships

Much research documents the importance of healthy relationships in extending the healthspan. For some, the use of The New Interpersonal Ethic may make or break the success of the hundred-year healthspan adventure. Recommendations are in Chapter 10.

These are the six components of the Healthspan System. When you use them, you will be bringing to each level of your Whole Self that quality of attention that promotes balance and harmony. As you have read and thought about using these six components, it may have occurred to you that this is a lot to do. In fact, you may be wondering how you could possibly do all this and still meet your other responsibilities and commitments. If so, I will address that good question in the next chapter.

Now that we have considered ways of giving a balancing quality of attention to each level of your Whole Self, let us turn to the equally important question of how to provide the appropriate quantity of attention.

The appropriate quantity of attention: giving priority to spirit

It is impossible to attain and maintain balance in the Whole Self if most of your attention is going to your body and little or none to your mind and spirit. The same is true for excessive attention to spirit to the neglect of body and mind, or to mind to the neglect of the spirit and the body. If your goal is to have reliable transportation, it is a mistake to get so preoccupied with keeping the proper pressure in the tires that you forget to refuel and change the oil. For example, not long ago I noticed a burning sensation in my left knee—an unusual occurrence. My joints, after 65 years of vigorous use, usually feel as good as they did when I was 24. I recognized the discomfort as a message from Mother Nature that something was out of balance. I began a survey of the levels of my Whole Self—and found something out of balance on *every* level.

On the body level, I had overstressed the knee while on a recent vacation by climbing too many mountains without proper conditioning. On the mind level, I had gotten so greedy for rapid progress on my part of this book that I had cut myself short of daily contact with Mother Nature and her healing energy. (She does not seem to hang around computers much.) On the level of the spirit, I had let that same greed result in my spending insufficient time each day in the experience of quiet alertness. This had deprived me of the healing energy and knowledge that knee and I needed from Spirit. The result: a knee that was saying, "Ouch!" Diagnosis done, I took the necessary action: spending more time outdoors in contact with nature and in quiet alertness. Within two days, the knee was saying, "Ah, I needed that!"

We have written at length about the power of attention. It is the power to create the life you want. Like time and energy, you have only a finite amount of attention to give. There is not enough to go around to everything you are interested in, much less to everything other people want you to be interested in. Therefore, you have to prioritize. You have to decide which things are important enough to get your attention and which ones are not—even though you may wish you had enough attention for them, too. Sometimes these are hard choices. The good can be the enemy of the best. You may sometimes have to sacrifice the good in order to have the best. The New Testament parable about the man who found hidden treasure in a field and sold everything he had to get money to buy the field is pertinent here. For help in making hard choices wisely, consider three operational principles: the Whole Self is a system, the higher in the system you work, the more leverage you have, and Spirit is very wise.

OPERATIONAL PRINCIPLES

OPERATIONAL PRINCIPLE 1: the Whole Self is a system

A system is a number of components so interconnected that changing one changes all. This is a factor that keeps the process of balancing the Whole Self from being impossibly complicated. Since you can change every level, at least somewhat, by changing one level, you do not have to work on every level all the time. Since some levels give you *much* more leverage than others, we will presently consider which is which. First, since the system concept is so powerful and important, consider an example of a system. I am fortunate to drive a Honda Civic, a well-engineered and competently constructed machine that has already given more years than I can remember of reliable service and shows no signs of quitting. In this vehicle, the power gets transferred from the engine to the front wheels through a series of gears that can be meshed, so that when one turns they all have to turn. If, at some day in the distant future, the starter will not work, I can start the engine by turning those gears. Theoretically, turning any gear in the system could do it, but it is easier to turn some than others. For example, since this Honda has a manual transmission, I could start it rolling downhill, then mesh the gears. Because they are a system, they all have to turn. Since one of them is connected to the engine, it has to turn, too. When it turns, it is most likely to start —and off we go. Theoretically, I could accomplish the same thing by turning the gear next to the one that is connected to the engine, but it is easier to turn the one connected to the wheels. This is the first factor that simplifies the balancing process; the second is the leverage factor.

OPERATIONAL PRINCIPLE 2: the leverage factor

Leverage is power or effectiveness gained from the mechanical advantage of using a lever. Archimedes, the great Greek mathematician, was so impressed with the power of leverage that he remarked, "Give me a place to rest my lever and I will move the world." When balancing the Whole Self, the higher in the system you work, the more leverage you have and the easier it is to balance the whole system. Look at the Whole Self Diagram. What is the highest level? Ah, Pure Consciousness! You have heard of that. That is the most efficient level at which to work, because creating balance there has an automatic balancing effect at every other level.

Now you have a clue about the mechanics that drive the remarkably favorable results on the mental and physical levels. Those results are now documented by dozens of research studies of the effects of meditation, the experience of quiet alertness.

Now, look at the bottom of the chart. There is the material level. That is where biochemistry is the operational principle. It is also the least efficient level at which to work to balance the Whole Self. Where do most people want to do their balancing work? Yep, on the biochemical level, with nutritional supplements, herbs, and the chemical cure of the month from *Prevention Magazine, The Ladies Home (Medical) Journal* and the two dozen throw-away publications that arrive in the mail each week.

Why do most people have it exactly backward—if they care about balance at all? There are many reasons, including, as Bob Dylan sang, "Money doesn't talk—it swears." People who make billions of dollars each year selling things that are supposed to improve health spend millions of those dollars on advertising. People who write the advertising copy are very good at what they do. What they intend to do is to convince you that matter matters most, that if you spend your money for this particular product, you have made your best investment in your health.

The best example I have seen recently is in a throwaway magazine about retarding aging. The front cover showed a picture of a woman's face. It had several large, brown age spots—not very attractive. The feature story said that age spots on the skin meant age spots in the brain. Age spots in the brain, according to this story, cause Alzheimer's. If you take the product, you can get rid of the brown age spots on your skin and in your brain, becoming beautiful and beating senility, all with one pill! Is it true? We do not know; we will wait until we read it from someone we trust. However, we do know it is effective advertising. Even I, who have been dropping such ads into trashcans for years, paused a moment before dropping this one. The millions spent on advertising play a part in the tendency to put the most emphasis on the lowest level of the Whole Self where it will do the least.

However, it is not only because of money and advertising, but also because of the superstition of materialism that most people go first to the level of matter and biochemistry. Remember Chapter Two? Yes, that was a long time and a lot of words ago. Let us refresh your memory. The superstition of materialism says, "If you cannot perceive it with one or more of your five senses, it is not real. If it is not real, you would be stupid to pay any attention to it."

With which of your five senses do you perceive the Field of Pure Consciousness? "See?" says the Superstition of Materialism; "It isn't real. Don't waste your time! Bop on down to the health food store or call this toll-free number for the Cure of the Month. You can see it and touch it. You may even be able to taste it and smell it. Therefore, it is real and worthy of your attention—and your money."

When you remember that we, as a culture, are just beginning to break free from this superstition, the surprising thing is not that most people go straight to the bottom of the diagram, to the material, least efficient level for balancing. The surprising thing is that so many are using meditation and other interventions, such as tai chi and yoga that work at higher, more efficient levels. It is like seeing a dog play checkers: the surprising thing is not that he plays badly, but that he plays at all.

Does this mean that one should work only on the Pure Consciousness level and ignore the rest, particularly the material level? Not at all! Sometimes, the material, biochemical level *should* be addressed first. There may be several reasons. The most important may be that the material level is where the individual's interest is. Of all the wonderful things our patients have taught us in the last 40 years, the most important is the Healthspan Center Principle: I *cannot treat the patient who is no longer here.*

If a new patient is interested in balancing her biochemistry and believes that is best done with nutritional supplements and maybe hormones, we had better talk supplements and hormones, or she will quickly find someone who will. Therefore, we do supplements and hormones. Then, after she is feeling better and we have gained some credibility with her, it may be time to talk about doing something higher up in the system. The opportunity usually presents, because no matter how much we fine-tune and tweak the supplements and hormones, no matter how much she improves, she will eventually realize that those things will not do all she wants done. Then she may be ready to hear about something more.

Another good reason to work on the biochemical level first is that the Whole Self may be so far out of balance as to put any other level temporarily out of reach. For example, a young woman, a freshman in college, consulted me about her depression. She was so depressed that she could not study or relate to her peers enough to form friendships. She felt panicky as she fell farther behind in academic work every day and she was very lonely. Depression, panic, and loneliness are an agonizing combination.

Her energy was so depleted and her cognitive function so impaired that it would have been futile to try to intervene above the material level without working there first. We found that she had a thyroid system disorder called Wilson's Syndrome. This condition, which is usually undetectable by blood tests, was slowing her metabolism to the point of depriving her of sufficient energy to function adequately physically and mentally. After supporting her thyroid system with the correct thyroid hormone, T-3, she felt and functioned better. Even so, she was still too depressed to address her main mental and spiritual issue: her purpose in life. She began supplementation with an amino acid derivative, phenylethylamine (PEA), which increases the effect of the neurotransmitter, norepinephrine. Some of the antidepressant drugs do that, too, but often at the price of troublesome side effects, including drowsiness.

She soon felt well enough to address her purpose in life issue. She entered cognitive-behavioral therapy and discovered that she had gone to an engineering school because her high school counselor and others had told her she was intelligent enough to do so. She had felt pressure from others and from her ego to attend a prestigious engineering school. She discovered through therapy that her purpose in life is to help other people through counseling, not through mechanical engineering. She changed schools and began to study psychology and art. For the first time in years, she began to experience happiness as she took action every day to fulfill her life purpose.

It is hard for us to imagine how she could have taken this difficult, decisive, effective action on the mental and spiritual levels of her Whole Self without the prior intervention on the physical level.

Sometimes, the process of helping a person balance her Whole Self is like digging out a pine tree stump. The stump will not come out until the taproot is cut, but the taproot cannot be cut first. One has to start at the surface, cut the feeder roots and throw them out of the hole, together with a lot of dirt, before he can cut the taproot and remove the stump. Even so, it is still true that the higher in the system you work, the more leverage you have. Let us now consider how to do that.

OPERATIONAL PRINCIPLE 3: Spirit is supremely wise.

Therefore, meet the energy and attention needs of your spirit first. Then you will find the wisdom to put the appropriate amount of attention and resources on every other level of your Whole Self. In *Sacred Verses, Healing Sounds*, Chopra said, "In the simplest terms, spirit is awareness." Since awareness is essential to any intelligent action, it seems reasonable to achieve an adequate amount of awareness before taking other action. "Look before you leap" is a succinct statement of this principle. "A shot in the dark" is an aphorism suggesting that the alternative is less skillful. Your spirit will tell you how much of your attention it needs. Let it speak to you through your heart.

Asking your heart for guidance on a complex and delicate issue may sound strange—and not very wise. As Chopra has observed, the heart has a reputation for being mushy and sentimental. He goes on to say, however, that this reputation in undeserved. In fact, the heart has a computing power far beyond that of the intellect. The most powerful intellect can consider a maximum of seven variables at once. That is to say, it can consider seven factors or aspects of a situation in an attempt to come to some conclusion about what to do.

The heart, according to Chopra, has the power of infinite correlation; that is, it can consider an infinite number of variables at once. I think this is because the heart is connected to the Cosmic Mainframe, which contains the data that runs the universe. In any case, the heart has a reputation for wisdom among the wise of the ages. In the Old Testament there is the scripture, "Keep your heart with all diligence, for out of it are the issues of life." Meher Baba, writing in this century, said, "The hidden depths of the ocean of life can be gauged only by sounding the heart." He also pointed out that knowledge of the intellect alone is on the same footing as mere information; and being superficial, moves on the surface of life. It gives the shadow and not the substance of reality. A practical aspect of this is that your heart knows what your spirit needs; your intellect does not—and probably does not care. If you choose to consult your heart on this vital matter, you may wish to have a technology for doing so.

Chopra's approach is to carefully notice what you feel in the area of your heart when you think about different options for accomplishing something. One choice will feel more comfortable around your heart than the others do. The feeling may be subtle, but it will be there. Once you sense that response, your heart has spoken. Select that option and, as Chopra says, "...plunge ahead with abandon." Another technology is to achieve the mind-state of quiet alertness, which gives you access to Pure Consciousness. The answer you seek is already in Pure Consciousness. When your attention goes there, your awareness expands there, and eventually you know what the answer is. Along with that knowing usually comes an experience of peace, joy, and certainty that you soon learn to realize is a confirmatory message from Pure Consciousness.

Cooperation between heart and intellect

In order for this process to work, the heart and the intellect must cooperate. Each has a vital function to perform. The heart decides what to do; the intellect decides how to do it. So long as the intellect keeps quiet until the heart has spoken, the process works smoothly. The problems arise if you do not make it clear to your intellect that it is to function in a tactical, not a strategic role. Most people's intellects are not accustomed to that. Instead, intellect is in the habit of figuring out what to do, and then how to do it. In our culture, intellect is encouraged to be arrogantly condescending to heart and to ruthlessly disregard its wisdom. Intellect may not take kindly to its new status, which it perceives as a demotion. It will probably try to continue deciding *what* as well as *how*. Nevertheless, you command your intellect and your heart through your attention. If you pay attention to your heart first, that is where your energy goes. Intellect then has no choice but to wait until you power it up by giving it your attention. That time comes when you need to select the route to the destination that your heart has chosen.

For example, a patient of mine suffers severely from chemical sensitivities. He has brain fog, depression, visual disturbances, memory lapses, and fatigue when he is exposed to chemicals in his workplace. He fears leaving his trade, which is the only way he knows to make a living. Anywhere he worked, there would be the same chemicals: they go with the territory. He felt trapped in misery by fear of worse misery. His suffering eventually escalated until he decided to listen to his heart, which said, "Leave your present employment." He decided to follow his heart. He then called on his intellect to find a way to carry out his decision. His intellect said, "You can go into business for yourself, doing what you know how to do and enjoy doing, and you can find a way to do it without the chemicals that are poisoning you. You can continue in your present employment for a few months while you save money and learn how to build cabinets and renovate houses without using toxic chemicals. There are many chemically sensitive people who will need your help in creating safe, less toxic living space."

He has begun to act on this plan. He has already enjoyed some decrease in his symptoms, although his chemical exposures have not yet decreased. He is better because he has created more balance and harmony on both the spirit and the mind levels of his Whole Self. Since the Whole Self is a system, more balance and harmony on the higher levels has brought more balance and harmony to the body level, including the biochemical, where the chemical sensitivity reactions occur.

This whole process of deciding how much attention to put where is made easier by the natural tendency of attention to go to the level of Whole Self where the need is greatest. Attention does not always do that, but it often does. In the Zen literature, there are many stories about the deaths of Zen masters. At the time of death, the entire essence of a lifetime of rigorous spiritual training and insight is often distilled and encapsulated in a death poem or a few last words. Because of this, the master's disciples gather at his deathbed in rapt attention and profound respect to hear his last communication to them. In one such instance, a disciple asked the dying master, "Where will you go, Master?"

"To hell," was the reply. Seeing the looks of horror and confusion on his disciple's faces, the master added, "Because that is where the need is greatest." Attention, like the Zen master, often goes to the place of greatest need. If you can recall hitting your thumb with a hammer, that experience will help you understand this principle.

The proof of the pudding

The final and conclusive piece of the technology is to put your plan into action and see what happens. Two things confirm the correctness of your choice: increasing comfort, particularly in your spirit, and synchronicities. Chopra has told us that nature sends us only two signals: comfort and discomfort. When we are moving into balance and harmony with nature, she sends the signal of comfort that says, "You made a good choice: Keep going." If she sends the signal of increasing discomfort that means, "Wait a minute! Something isn't working here. Review the process and see what's wrong." This does not mean that there will be a steady, constant increase in comfort so long as you are on the right track. You may be exactly on course, but have some very uncomfortable days or weeks, due to complications of karma and other factors. However, if you use a longer time frame, a month or quarters of years, you can usually detect a growing experience of comfort, particularly in the area of your heart. If there is increasing discomfort there, that is an unequivocal warning to reevaluate, no matter how comfortable body and mind may be.

Consider, for example, a situation in which you might be running from a hungry bear. You are running for your life, at top speed. Your heart is pounding, your lungs feel as if they are bursting, your legs seem to be on fire, and you are terrified. You are anything but comfortable in several ways. If, however, every time you look back, you see the distance between you and the bear increasing, you get a certain unmistakable feeling of increased comfort. Sometimes, when you are acting on your heart's decision, it is like that. The final confirmation of the correctness of your choice comes only from acting on it. So long as you only think about it, you will never know.

STRATEGIC PRINCIPLE 3: deal with the problems of ego and karma

There are two problems, ego and karma, that specifically need to be addressed in forming and executing your strategy. Here is a discussion of these problems and some suggestions for dealing with them.

The problem of karma

Karma is a term for the law of cause and effect, particularly cause and effect on the moral plane. It is increasingly recognized as a major force in determining what people experience in their lives. The wisdom traditions of the East, Vedic and Buddhism, consider it a major determinant of human happiness and suffering. In the Christian tradition, the law of karma is summarized in the verse, "Be not deceived, God is not mocked. Whatsoever you sow that shall you also reap. If you sow to the flesh, from the flesh you will reap corruption. If you sow to the spirit, from the spirit, you will reap everlasting life."

I have already written about the most painful experience in my life: Andy's death. The law of karma was a major factor in that experience. Years earlier, I had set in motion forces that at a particular point in time produced results that were extremely painful. Although I was experiencing severe suffering, I was extraordinarily fortunate in understanding that I had caused the pain. My Zen teacher, Roshi Philip Kapleau, was a great benefactor when he said, "The answer to the question, what did I do to deserve this? is always, 'Plenty!'" Before I heard that, I had lived by the principle, "To err is human; to find someone to blame it on is genius." Had I still been doing that, the outcome of the excruciatingly painful experience of Andy's death would have been different, and it is unlikely that any good would have come of it. As it was, since I knew that I was reaping the karmic consequences of my own behavior, I did not have to waste energy blaming other people or trying to punish them for my suffering. I was free to use what energy I had to read the message in the catastrophe and see the opportunities that were hidden in all that pain and danger. Because I was free to do this, I was able to use suffering to power a quantum jump to a higher level in the practice of holistic medicine. Understanding the law of karma brings the benefit of being able to focus energy and attention on finding the solutions to the problems rather than wasting it on blaming others or trying to get revenge, in the process creating many more problems.

There is another reason that the understanding of the law of karma and how to use it to your advantage is crucially important. If you understand this law, you are much less likely to get discouraged and give up if you do not immediately feel better when you apply the principles that you are now learning. It may be that you are doing exactly the thing you need to do in order to achieve your 100-year healthspan. You may not be feeling better yet because some heavy karma has ripened and must be worn out before you can feel the benefit of what you have begun to do.

There are two kinds of karma: favorable and heavy. There is no problem with favorable karma, as long as you understand that you are having a pleasant or favorable experience because you did something helpful or beneficial for someone or something at some time in the past. It is important to understand two other things about karma. The first is that all karma, favorable or heavy, eventually wears out. The second is that you are creating new karma all the time, until you learn how to act without creating any. Once you get tired of karma and really want to free yourself from it forever, you can learn how to do that. A good way to start is by listening to Chopra's commentary on the *Bhagavad Gita* in his album, *Sacred Verses, Healing Sounds*.

Freeing yourself from karma is another story for another time, but it is worth mentioning here because it can be done; the protocol for doing it has been clearly described and available for about five thousand years. You must do it to finally get free from suffering. In the meantime, you are always having both favorable and heavy karma ripening and making its influence felt in your life. The challenge is to deal skillfully with heavy or painful karma.

In *The Seven Spiritual Laws of Success*, there is an important discussion of how to deal with heavy karma. Briefly stated, Chopra recommends three approaches: gradually washing the karma away by daily meditation, paying the karmic debt, and transforming the karma with a more desirable experience. He then gives instructions about how to do all this. Since all of us have heavy karma ripening from time to time, this skill is valuable for claiming birthrights, to say nothing of reducing suffering. Zen teaching, as well as Chopra's writings, emphasizes the value of meditation for lightening heavy karma. In a Zen chant there is the line, "Thus one true samadhi (a very deep state of meditation) extinguishes evils; it purifies karma, dissolving obstructions."

Another useful Zen principle is that when something painful happens, place your hands together palm to palm and give thanks to your Higher Power that you are being allowed to pay a karmic debt sooner, while it is lighter, rather than later when it would be heavier. It is hard to remember to do this when something painful or disturbing is happening, but when you do it, you will notice a surprisingly beneficial effect on the pain and the disturbance.

Finally, Chopra recommends finding a way to turn the painful experience into a beneficial one for you and for others. This actually happened in several of the experiences I have written about: my destruction of my medical practice, Andy's death, and losses in the flood.

In summary, once you gain some understanding of the law of karma you will suffer much less when heavy karma ripens and manifests in your life. You are more likely to turn the painful experience into a beneficial one for you and for others. You are more likely to persist with your 100-year healthspan program, instead of giving up when you do not see immediate results. Persistence will enable you to win one of the most wonderful, delightful, joyful experiences of your entire life.

The Problem of ego

Ego is the other problem that must be understood and solved, at least partially, in order to achieve the 100-year healthspan. Having discussed the problem of ego in Chapter 8, we will summarize briefly here. Then I will offer suggestions about how to solve the ego problem.

Ego is a necessary evil during part of the long journey to full realization of Pure Consciousness. Ego is necessary because of the Mistake of the Intellect, discussed in Chapter 4. Due to the Mistake of the Intellect, life appears to be made up of a bewildering array of unconnected experiences, objects, and sensations. The ego emerges as part of the attempt to make sense of, organize, and manage what appears to be overwhelming diversity.

The attempt succeeds reasonably well, but at an exorbitant price. The price is that your ego develops the false idea that you are your body. This creates the illusion of separateness and division between internal and external life. Since the ego is based on the illusion of separateness instead of the reality of the oneness of all life, it is the source of unending trouble. It consistently mistakes the important for the unimportant, and vice versa.

Since it is founded on a false idea, it is forever insecure and uneasy. It tries to feel secure by amassing material possessions and power. Since this desperate struggle is foredoomed to failure, ego has incurable *more* disease: whatever you have, it demands more. Being incapable of satisfaction, it is usually irritable, frustrated, and contentious. This basic orientation to life creates a level of stress, confusion, and anxiety that is hostile to much of life—and especially to the 100-year healthspan. This is why the ego problem must be solved, at least partially, if you are to claim your birthright from nature.

Meher Baba describes the best system that I know for solving the ego problem. It begins with the procedure for sabotaging the ego, an adaptation of which I described in Chapter 8, in the section on Sabotaging the Saboteur. It takes the process one step further, to create a new provisional ego, serving the purpose of organizing and managing experience, but free of the fatal mistake of the original ego.

The additional step flows naturally from the preceding ones. As review, they are:

1. Focus your attention constantly on your Higher Power.

2. Cultivate deep, intense love for your Higher Power.

3. Express that love by doing what your Higher Power wishes you to do in each situation you encounter.

4. Make what you have done a gift of love to your Higher Power, forget it, and go on to the next thing.

5. Each time you do this, ego becomes weaker, love for your Higher Power becomes stronger, and your power to do what your Higher Power wishes done increases.

The additional step is:

As your attention goes more and more to your Higher Power, "where attention goes, energy flows." It flows away from your ego, which becomes weaker. It flows into your awareness of your Higher Power, which becomes stronger. In this way, Your Higher Power becomes your provisional ego, serving the organizing function better than the original, and free of the fatal flaw.

Since your Higher Power is the embodiment and source of the oneness of all life, you now have the perfect antidote to the mistake of the ego, the false idea that you are your physical body and separate from everything else in the universe.

In other words, the provisional ego gets the job done better, without causing trouble in the process. This minimizes stress, confusion, and trouble that are such deadly enemies of the 100-year healthspan. It maximizes joy, power, fun, fellowship, and fulfillment that are such powerful facilitators of that healthspan.

STRATEGIC PRINCIPLE 4: strategic planning

Once your heart has spoken and you have set your intellect to the task of deciding how to execute heart's strategy, intellect may tell you that there is no way to get there from here. What heart has decided is necessary, intellect considers impossible. In the case of the cabinetmaker, intellect concluded that it was impossible to make an acceptable and predictable living without exposure to toxic chemicals. Whenever intellect says this, what it means is, "This change is impossible right now." The heart can always see farther than the intellect—and larger, too. The big picture that the heart sees may actually take months, and sometimes years, to paint. Neither you nor your intellect need be daunted at this. To be on your way to the 100-year healthspan, you do not have to arrive at the destination heart has selected; you only have to be on the way. As soon as you commit to following your heart's orders, a number of favorable things start to happen. You discover the first step in the process. When you take that step, you see the next one. The synchronicities start. Health and energy improve. As Thoreau said, you begin to "...meet with a success unexpected in common hours."

The crucial thing is to take action every day to move toward your goal, no matter how far away it seems. Every single day will, in fact, bring something you can do to move. Most days will bring more to do than you can get around to. You will discover the truth of the sayings, "The road is better than the inn," and "Life is a journey, not a destination." There is always a freedom and freshness in this way of being. There is no stagnation and you never get trapped.

Happiness is not a station you arrive at, but a manner of traveling.

—Margaret Lee Runbeck

Chapter 14

BALANCING WHOLE SELF: TACTICS

A TACTICAL TRIUMPH

When Dale first entered my consulting room, I thought she was one of a seemingly endless procession of depressed women who sought treatment at the mental health center. She was pale, deeply depressed, and looked anguished. I assumed that this would be another consultation like the dozen or two new patient visits I had already done that week. Then I noticed her eyes. They had the desperate, pleading expression of a drowning person going down for the third time. Then I thought I saw something else: a faint flicker of determination to do something—perhaps to regain her health. Suddenly she had my heightened attention; something extraordinary was going on here.

I took her history. She was a teacher, working until a few weeks before, when she was disabled by a manic episode of bipolar (manic-depressive) disorder. After she spent a few days in a hospital, her condition stabilized enough to permit her discharge and return home to continue her recovery. She was consulting me after she had been at home for about three weeks. In the meantime, she had cycled from mania to depression. Thorazine, which had helped to control mania, was making her depression worse.

I began to taper her Thorazine and to cautiously treat her with an antidepressant, hoping that it would not push her into another manic state. She was already taking lithium as a mood stabilizer; we continued that. Gradually, her depression decreased and she regained emotional and mental freedom to function as we reduced and then discontinued Thorazine. I learned that the most horrible part of the experience had been her inability, mostly due to the Thorazine, to think and to feel. She had a keen intellect and an intense love for using it to learn and to teach. To have it blunted and constricted by medications was torture to her. She also had an unusually high level of awareness, which enabled her to experience more of everything than most people do. Losing that expansive awareness had been, if anything, worse than the impairment of her intellect. When she began to regain access to both, she was much relieved and very grateful.

Within two months, it was clear that she was in a stable remission. We began to discuss tactics for protecting her from another devastating mania or depression. The safest course is usually to continue lithium or one of the other mood stabilizing drugs indefinitely. The majority of patients with bipolar disorder relapse within a few months of discontinuing mood stabilizers. Since each relapse tends to be more severe and prolonged, it is urgently important to prevent them. As we discussed this, it became clear that indefinitely taking any kind of medication to stabilize mood was unacceptable to Dale. Although lithium was far less impairing to her thinking and feeling than Thorazine, she was unwilling to accept even that level of dulling. Like most people with bipolar disorder, she grossly underestimated the risk and danger of relapse. At the same time, she trusted me enough to be willing to try to work out a mutually agreeable balance between safety and freedom.

I recommended a Healthspan program similar to the one in the preceding chapter. As usual, meditation was the key. I taught her how to do Zen meditation, which she practiced as though her life depended on it. On the biochemical level, she soon learned which foods agreed with her and which did not. I think she was in the top five percent of my patients in conscientious adherence to a wholesome diet. We devised a nutritional supplementation program featuring large doses of B vitamins and vitamin C. Her most important energy intervention was regular physical exercise. She loved to swim and was resourceful in finding places where she could swim for an hour or more each day, summer and winter. Another crucial part of her recovery strategy was to balance activity and stillness. This was a challenge for her because she passionately loved teaching and she was working on a postgraduate degree. She was constantly tempted to over-schedule and overcommit to intense mental activity. She was spending at least half an hour twice a day in the deep stillness of meditation. She soon learned how much activity she could tolerate during the rest of the day. When she exceeded that limit, she either had to increase her meditation time or begin to slide back into mania.

As the months came and went, I began to understand that she was executing the tactics of her recovery program more completely than any other patient that I had ever treated. That faint flicker of determination to be healthy, that I thought I had glimpsed in the first consultation, now burned as a steady flame. Still, neither of us knew how much protection this masterful execution of the tactics of her holistic recovery program would give her against another devastating relapse into bipolar illness. She continued implacable in her determination to live drug-free, so we agreed on a gradual reduction in her drugs, first the antidepressant, then the lithium. Eventually, she was drug-free. I began a relapse vigil. Three months passed, then six, then nine. Most patients would have relapsed by then; Dale did not. After a drug-free year, I knew that something unusual was going on.

Her second year was nearly drug free. Once during that year, she found herself in an overstress situation from which she could find no immediate escape. No amount of meditation and increased exercise would stabilize her. She agreed to resume lithium, but took it for only a few weeks, until she could get her life rebalanced. In the 10 years that have elapsed since then, she has occasionally taken small doses of lithium for a few days at a time while she was dealing with unusually high stress. She has always responded to one fourth to one half of the usual treatment dose.

In a recent followup visit (I now see her about once a year) she said, "I have learned that I have to do *all* of my recovery program every day. If I let any of it slip, I'm in trouble within a day or two." Dale does not feel burdened or oppressed by the necessity of such impeccable tactical execution. She remembers the horror of losing control of her mind and emotions and the suffocating mental and spiritual dulling by the medications. She is joyful that she has found a natural way to stay free of both bipolar disorder and drugs. She cherishes her freedom to use her keen intellect and exquisitely high level of awareness to learn and to teach in her field of interest. This fulfills her life mission, so it is a source of durable joy to her.

I have never known another patient to do what Dale has done. Most of my bipolar patients can not even imagine exercising the degree of self-discipline that Dale practices every day. Most of them quit taking their drugs after being in remission for a few weeks or months, then relapse into a longer, more severe manic or depressive episode. I hesitated to include Dale's story in this book, because some people with bipolar disorder will use it an excuse to quit taking their medications. I decided to write it anyway for two reasons. First, tens of thousands of people with bipolar disorder have found some excuse to stop medications. None of them ever heard of Dale and her remarkable achievement. Second, people who have bipolar disorder need to know Dale's story.

Most of my bipolar patients ask me if there is an alternative to taking mood stabilizers indefinitely. They, and hundreds of thousands of others, need to know that, with sound strategy and impeccable tactics, it *may* be possible to live free of drugs and bipolar disorder at the same time. Many more people need the encouragement of such a brilliant example of the power of the conscientious, consistent execution of a comprehensive tactical approach to the 100-year healthspan. To those people who have bipolar disorder and read this, I say, *"Please do not stop taking your prescribed medications until you do so with the agreement of a knowledgeable physician and until you have in operation a tactical program of this quality and consistency."*

CREATING YOUR ACTION PLAN

Most of this book is about how to achieve balance and harmony. There is so much knowledge, and there are so many things that you *could* do, that you might feel confused, even overwhelmed, at first. In this chapter, we are offering detailed instructions on how to sort it all out and create the healthspan program that works best for you in your unique situation now. In this section, I will tell you the six things that will, in my experience, probably be most important for empowering you to claim your birthright. This short list is the best of the best of what I have learned in over 40 years of medical practice. I will give the interventions in the order of their importance to most people. However, each person is unique: this priority list may not be right for you. As we are about to discuss, the most important thing is to start where you are; that is, *start with what interests you most.*

Start where you are! Your Healthspan program will result in your gaining the power to balance your Whole Self: your mind, your body, and your spirit. Since you cannot learn to do all three at once, your first decision is where to start. The key here is to start where you are. That means to start where your interest is and with what is feasible for you. Think back over the Healthspan Program and the chapters on The Power of Attention, Who Am I, Why Am I Here, Who Are All These Others, Balancing Energy, and Balancing Biochemistry. Notice which one draws your interest most strongly. That is where you are and that is where you can best begin.

If you feel about equally interested in working on each of these levels, start with quiet alertness and strengthening your power of attention. This is wise because, as previously noted, the whole flow of the universe is from consciousness to matter, from mind to molecules. If you balance consciousness first, then your balanced consciousness will have a balancing effect on your body (energy and biochemistry) and on your mind. It will also sharpen your intuition about what to do next. This will make everything you do on the mental and physical levels easier and quicker.

Set your pace. Decide how fast you want to reach your goals—and how much time, energy, and money you are willing to invest in doing it. Think about this analogy. Several people are climbing a mountain in order to enjoy a spectacular view from the top. Some of them are so eager to get there that they run up the mountain. They reach the summit first, sweating, panting, and weary. Others do not care for such extreme exertion. They climb slowly, with frequent rest stops. By the time they arrive, the first group has been enjoying the view and the breeze for some time. The remainder of the group ascends at a rate somewhere between the two extremes. So it is with those who set out to attain the 100-year healthspan. Each individual finds his or her own balance between comfort and speed.

In practical terms, there are decisions about how much time, energy, money, and attention you will invest. Perhaps the time commitment is the easiest to quantify. Decide how many minutes per day you will invest.

Here are the priorities I suggest for daily time commitments from 15 to 110 minutes per day.

15: Quiet Alertness

30: Quiet Alertness and the Five Rites of Rejuvenation

45: Quiet Alertness, the Five Rites of Rejuvenation, and 15 minutes of physical exercise

60: Quiet Alertness for 20 minutes, the Five Rites of Rejuvenation, and 20 minutes of physical exercise

75: Quiet Alertness for 20 minutes, the Five Rites of Rejuvenation, and 30 minutes of physical exercise

90: Quiet Alertness for 20 minutes, the Five Rites of Rejuvenation, and 45 minutes of physical exercise

110: Quiet Alertness for 20 minutes twice daily, the Five Rites of Rejuvenation, and 45 minutes of physical exercise

These things take the most time. Others, like eating a wholesome diet, do not take significantly longer, once you know how, than eating a disease diet. Nor does it take long to swallow the supplements recommended in the Healthspan Program.

Here are a few more tips. If you do something every day for a month, you own it; it becomes part of your lifestyle. When that happens, it takes less energy to continue doing it. Where your birthright program is concerned, this means that you can continue what you have been doing with less energy expenditure. Then, you have some energy left over to begin another component of your program with no additional energy drain.

In fact, you will have an energy gain, because each component you add increases your available energy. It does so in several ways. First, it gets you connected with the inexhaustible source of energy that runs the universe. Second, it reduces the energy you waste doing things that do not contribute to your 100-year healthspan or to the fulfillment of your purpose in life. Third, your body's ability to generate energy is increased by the more favorable biochemical and energy balance that you are gaining. Increasing energy empowers you to add components to your Healthspan program.

We have seen people get excited about many things, but the most delightedly excited people we ever see are those who are taking action every day to claim and enjoy their birthright. You have read an example in the preceding chapter in the excerpts from the journal of a woman who has had the experience. Part of the delight and excitement comes from being in the process of fulfilling the purpose for which they came into this life, a process that is the only reliable source of lasting happiness. This wonderful synergy of delight, excitement, wonder, awe, and achievement is part of nature's birthright to you. Watch for it, enjoy it, and let it be your assurance that you are doing the right thing at the right time at the right pace.

100 Days for 100 Years

Would you like to invest 100 days to create a lifestyle that is probably going to increase the quality, satisfaction, fun, and fulfillment of your life every day from now until you are 100? You would not have to quit work, leave your family, or go to some far-away place. You may even be able to make this investment with some of the time you now spend watching TV. If 100 days for 100 years sounds like a good deal, here is how you could do it, week by week.

Week 1:

a) Begin to practice quiet alertness (Chapter 5).

b) Order the *Five Rites of Rejuvenation* video and *The Eye of Revelation*, so that they will be available by the time you are ready to start doing them (Chapter 11)

c) Begin taking Basic Preventive 3 or 5. (Chapter 12)

Week 2:

a) Add the chi gong part of the Flick Protocol. (Chapter 11)

b) Start reading *The Zone*. (Chapter 12)

c) Begin the Ascorbate Protocol (Appendix)

Week 3:

a) Add walking, swimming, or an equivalent exercise. (Chapter 11)

b) Order a flax seed meal kit or start taking flax seed oil. (Chapter 12) If you order the kit, start using it as soon as it arrives.

Week 4:
Begin taking calcium citrate 500 mg twice daily with food. (Chapter 12)

Week 5:
a) Begin the Zone diet (Chapter 12)

b) Begin vitamin E (mixed tocopherols) 400 U twice daily. (Chapter 12)

Week 6:
a) Begin the Five Rites of Rejuvenation. (Chapter 11)

b) Begin vitamin D 400 U twice daily

Weeks 7 & 8:
Write your personal mission statement. (Chapter 9)

Weeks 9 & 10:
Read *The Celestine Vision*. Begin practicing The New Interpersonal Ethic (Chapter 10)

Week 11:
Do the first clearing ritual for your family tree. (Chapter 11)

Weeks 12 through 14:
Catch up on anything you have not gotten done yet, fine tune, troubleshoot, and enjoy. By now, you will probably be pleased at how much better you are feeling and functioning—and at the quality of adventure and fulfillment your life has taken on.

If you do not do all these things, no problem. If you even do one, you will benefit. If you do more than one, the synergy starts to work for you, and you will probably want to add more as you go along. The feeling of growing, glowing health gets addictive: you want more and more.

Make your commitment

As soon as you decide what you will do when, write out your agenda and sign it. Tell no one what you have decided, unless you are certain that he or she will be supportive. Friends and family, particularly family, will probably try to keep you doing things the way they are accustomed to, even when it seems obvious that you and they will benefit from your new plan. It is a curious characteristic of emotional systems, such as families, that they try to maintain sameness. Nothing personal—just the way emotional systems work. Nevertheless, you do not need other people siding with your ego against your 100-year healthspan program, so hold your cards close to your chest. Once you have made an intervention, such as meditation, part of your lifestyle, it will be a good idea to tell people who are close to you why you did it. Be prepared to have some of them try to get you to stop doing it. Do not worry; still nothing personal, just emotional systems at work. Simply keep on doing it. Some day, maybe years later, you may hear the other person say that starting to meditate was the best thing you ever did. It really does not matter whether or not they do: you will *know* it is one of the best things that you ever did.

There are some things, such as changing your diet, that you may need help with. Be careful here: there are three things that are such emotional issues that few people can be rational about them. Those things are religion, politics—and food. If someone else at home prepares your food, be as casual as you can about requesting some changes. Just mention that you have been reading about some foods that will help you feel better and that you would like to try some of them.

Keep a journal. As you begin this adventure, start a journal. On the first page, write your commitment and date and sign it. This increases your power to keep it. Make daily notes about what you experience while carrying out your program. Be careful to note all favorable experiences you have. Include any synchronicities ("fortunate coincidences") that you notice. You will, in fact, notice an increase in these fortunate coincidences, which really are not coincidences at all. They are evidence that you are moving yourself more into balance and harmony with the energy and intelligence that operates the universe. The more balance and harmony you achieve, the more support you get from this energy and intelligence. You will become increasingly convinced that they are much more than random chance. You will come to know that there is a master intelligence guiding your life, along with the rest of the universe, and that this powerful intelligence is arranging unsuspected and sometimes breathtakingly effective help for you as you go forward with the fulfillment of your life. It is empowering, energizing, and inspiring to be able to read back through your journal and remind yourself of these occurrences.

You should set aside ten or fifteen minutes once a week to review your journal, see what you have learned from the experiences of the past week, and then write a preview of the most important things you intend to do and experience in the coming week. Sunday is a good day for most people to do this, but the important thing is that you do it, not when you do it. If you, like most people, watch a good bit of television, taking fifteen minutes away from TV viewing to invest in journal writing and reviewing is an extraordinarily powerful balancing procedure for you.

Make midcourse adjustments. Life is dynamic and ever changing. Even the most perfect strategy and tactics need to be revised to respond to changing conditions. The same principles and practices you used to create your 100-year healthspan program will work when you sense that it needs to be adjusted. If it quits being fun and an adventure, it does need adjustment!

Enjoy the adventure; keep it fun! The key here is to keep it fun. When I started practicing holistic medicine, one of the most surprising things I heard was "This is fun!" By then I had practiced medicine for 25 years without ever hearing a patient say that anything I prescribed was fun. Now that I am doing holistic medicine, I have heard it more than once. The patients who say it are the ones who make the best and fastest progress. I think that is because they are implementing their programs in a way that maintains balance with the other things they are doing in their lives. I see some patients get excited when they hear about the Healthspan Program—and try to do it all at once. They rapidly get bogged down, overburdened, and overwhelmed. The whole process becomes anything but fun, so they soon abandon it.

If it *was* fun and you notice that it is not fun anymore, consider simplifying. Thoreau said that the three rules for successful living are *simplify, simplify, simplify*. I call it doing less better, rather than more worse. Scale back your program, rather than abandoning it.

The one thing that helps most in keeping the Healthspan program fun is finding other people who are doing it or something similar. If you persist with the program, you will find them. You will find them sooner if you are practicing the New Interpersonal Ethic. If, in addition, you are in the process of fulfilling your purpose, you will find them even sooner.

You now have an understanding of the strategy and tactics for going on the greatest adventure of your life. If you do not already feel the excitement of this adventure, you will when the experiences and results begin to flow into your life! Persist in the process you have begun. You are likely to discover what Tagore, the Indian Nobel Laureate in Poetry, meant when he wrote, "The heaven's river has drowned its banks and the flood of joy is abroad."

Epilogue

GRACEFUL EXITS

Everybody has to die of something.

Dr. Jeffrey Bland, the foremost innovator and educator in the field of functional medicine, told of a participant in one of his seminars who made the above remark, apparently questioning the value of using the health enhancing modalities that Dr. Bland was teaching. Bland responded that not everybody has to start the decline in their 40's or 50's. He amplified the point with the following story about his grandfather.

Grandfather, at the age of ninety-six, enjoyed playing marathon canasta games with the rest of the family. He was lively and active. When he was in his eighties he was demonstrating to his grandchildren how to do handsprings and handstands. During a canasta marathon, he told the other family members that this would be his last one. He said that he had lived a long time, had enjoyed seeing his grandchildren grow up and now he was ready to move on. He died a few weeks later, without being sick or experiencing any trauma. He just decided it was time for a transition and he made it in his own way and in his own time.

While it may be true that everyone has to die of something, Jeff's grandfather demonstrated that it does not have to be illness, disease, or trauma. Some people apparently die of having completed what they came into this life to do. It is not unusual for those individuals to die with a deep serenity and sense of fulfillment. The Chinese say of such a person, "He has eaten." An old song says, "But one thing I know, when it comes my time, I'll leave this old world with a satisfied mind."

The following stories show that Jeff's grandfather was not unique in his high attainment.

I was sitting on the treatment table with two electrodes on my neck. There was a faint tingling sensation as Carl, my chiropractor, applied micro-current to accelerate the healing of an old whiplash injury that had been aggravated by excessive use of force with a pickaxe in hard clay. As we waited for the clock to run on the micro-current treatment, we were talking about the hundred-year healthspan. Carl was saying, "When my grand-daddy was ninety-four, he used to walk five miles around his farm every morning. It was during the depression in the thirties, and most of the family had come back home to the farm because there was food there. One day when grandpa returned from his walk, the family was gathering for dinner. He said to some of the grandchildren, 'I have lived a long time. I have made a lot of money; I have seen everything I want to see and done everything I want to do, so today I think I'll die.'"

"The grandchildren thought he was teasing them. They said, 'Aw, grandpa, you're ninety-four years old. You're going to live till you're more than a hundred.'

"Grandpa went out on the front porch and sat in a rocker. When someone went to call him to dinner, he didn't respond. Nobody could get him to respond. Someone called the family doctor who came and gave him a shot. When he still did not respond the doctor pronounced him dead."

I said to Carl, "A death such as the one you have just described to me seems to me to be evidence of a high level of spiritual development."

He agreed.

The director of a mental health center told me that her grandfather had told his wife during planting season that he was ready to die, except that he wanted to make one more crop for her and their son. He continued to farm as usual throughout the summer, then harvested the crop. On the day he completed the harvest, he ate a large dinner, lay down, and died.

Jack Derby, inventor of a violet ray healing device, said that it is the divine plan for humans to live completely healthy lives and die with a perfectly healthy body. Remember Dr. Chopra's definition of perfect health: a preponderance of bliss over discomfort. I agree with both Derby and Chopra. You have just read some stories that support this contention.

The Zen literature abounds in wonderful accounts of the deaths of the Zen masters. One of them is about Hue Neng, the sixth patriarch of Zen. On the first of June, he told his disciples that he would die on June 30. Since he went about his business as usual, they thought that he was teasing him and were not concerned. On June 30th, the patriarch put on his ceremonial robes and sat meditation until he toppled over dead.

When a modern Zen master was dying, one of his disciples spent the day searching the pastry shops of Tokyo for a confection the master particularly enjoyed. He finally found it and rushed back to the monastery to find that the master was weakening rapidly and death was imminent. He presented the confection to the master who took a bite and ate it. He then appeared very near death. His disciples leaned toward him intently, begging him to give them his final words. He said, "My! But that cake was delicious." With that, he died.

Henry David Thoreau said many inspiring, helpful, and memorable things, but none more so than his remark to his aunt who visited him when he was on his deathbed. She asked, "Henry, have you made your peace with God?"

Thoreau replied, "We never quarreled."

In the Indian culture, death is sometimes referred to as "dropping the body." For one who understands that the Higher Self is imperishable and immortal, while only the body perishes, this Indian expression is more accurate than the Western term, dying. Meher Baba wrote that most of the horror many people feel about death is due to the mistaken belief that the person is the physical body. Here the superstition of materialism takes a heavy toll. Once one realizes, "I am *not* my body; I am infinite and eternal," the fear and dread of death loosens its grip. This liberating realization comes with the repeated experience of the Higher Self, made possible by the mind-state of quiet alertness.

Consider an analogy from the space program. There comes a time in a space mission when the commander of the space shuttle separates the shuttle from the booster rocket, which then falls to its destruction, having served its purpose. The shuttle continues its mission unencumbered, eventually to be fitted with another booster for another mission.

Much has been written about the value and desirability of a "conscious death." Not everyone appreciates that. Woody Allen has been quoted as saying; "I don't mind dying. I just don't want to be there when it happens." Those who are still trapped in the superstition of materialism may be mystified about anyone wanting to be conscious in order to lose consciousness in death. Accumulating evidence suggests that the apparent loss of consciousness is part of the superstition of materialism. The actual experience seems more likely to be an expansion of consciousness. All reports of the near death experiences support this probability. Most of the great religions include it as part of their teaching.

In Buddhist teaching it is suggested that the benefit of a conscious death is a higher level of consciousness in one's next existence. "The last thought in the previous existence is the first thought in the next existence." Zen teacher Philip Kapleau has written a book, *The Wheel of Life and Death*. It is a rich resource for the technology of achieving a desirable, conscious death and for nurturing others who wish to do so. Such a transition is a magnificent and fitting culmination of nature's birthright to humans, the 100-year healthspan.

STAY TUNED: THE BEST IS YET TO COME!

Body getting older, mind getting newer,
Like flint against steel, opposite hard thrust.
Shower of sparks lights up the Void,
Starts growing flames in tinder minds.

—OJW

Healthspan is an introduction to a vast, rapidly expanding, and evolving body of knowledge of how to claim your human birthright from nature. In this book, there is plenty of knowledge for you to use to get started, but there is far more knowledge than you may wish to use to claim and enjoy your birthright fully. We intend to bring forward much more of this knowledge in subsequent books. Genevieve is preparing to write *Living Love: Love and Relationships for Your 100-Year Healthspan.* I have begun work on *Crisis Mastery: a holistic approach to Y2K and other complex systems failures.* If the computer still works after 1 January, I expect to write *The 100-Year Healthspan for Folks Over 50.* Beyond that, we have several other books in mind, but the knowledge base is expanding so fast as to make it impossible to predict what area will demand our attention after we send these next two to the printer. We intend to be writing, publishing, and giving workshops, seminars, and lectures until we have used up our entire 100-year healthspans. For updates on new information we have for you, visit our home page, www.healthspirit.com.

I know what happiness is, for I have done good work.

—Robert Lewis Stevenson

Appendix

CLEARING FOR THE FAMILY TREE

This document is part of a manuscript being prepared for publication by Denny Ray Johnson. I am grateful for his generosity in permitting me to present it here.

—OJW

Prayer is God's gift to all of us. Regardless of your religion, prayer is always available to you. Prayer is universal and its deeper mysteries will be forever beyond the full comprehension of mankind. As man evolves, the richness of prayer will increase, in accordance with the nature of the divine. Prayer does not require a religion, only a sincere heart and love for God. And prayer does not require that you understand how the higher levels work. All that is required is that you do your heartfelt best to focus your mind and allow the higher levels to work.

Prayer is like a tool in the hands of a doctor, and it is wise to understand when and how to use it. Learning to improve your use of prayer is a life-long lesson. Prayer does not replace a medical doctor or good counselor, and physical and mental symptoms are largely our responsibility, to be dealt with appropriately.

Spiritual issues belong to the spiritual world, and prayer does not pound nails into wood or put a wet cloth on the fevered brow of a sick child. Prayer does not put a spoonful of chicken soup into someone's mouth, nor does it replace the loving hand of a mother. Prayer has a specific purpose; it works primarily in the spiritual realms. Although it does affect physical matter and mental problems, it starts within spirit, and extends beyond matter and mind. Prayer is timeless, transcending generations.

If you see a recurring problem in your family, such as anger or alcoholism, it is important to realize that the problem did not begin in your immediate family. It is not solely the result of how that person was treated as a child. In fact, nothing of true consequence started in any one person's childhood. It was carried forward from somewhere else in the family tree. Anger or alcoholism that has gone on for more than three generations is no longer just a physical or psychological problem. It has become the spirit of anger or the spirit of alcoholism that torments the family. The same is true of other forms of addictive behavior such as jealousy, racism, criticism, sexual violence, and hate. No allopathic or naturopathic medicines will work at this level. In such cases, the family needs help from the spiritual realms of light and love.

When you ask the spiritual realms for help, follow the principles of your own religion. Apply what you hold to be true about the power of prayer. Do it in your own way or follow someone you trust. Ask for guidance from a spiritual counselor within your faith, or from the wisest grandparent you can find. From experience, they should know what to do. If you have doubts, consider these simple guidelines.

1. Acknowledge that it is the higher levels that are doing the work.

2. Focus your attention on the family line where you believe the spirit of the difficulty originates.

3. Come from your heart, and speak your prayer aloud.

4. Give thanks for the blessings and gifts these difficulties have brought to your family.

5. Pray again for the spiritual strengths within the family lines (where once you saw difficulty) to now be brought forth.

6. Repeat the prayer about once a month for four months.

As a grandparent, focus your prayer first on the four generations that came before you, even if you did not know them. Then focus your prayer on the four generations coming after you, even if they are not yet conceived. Be a good grandparent. Take a few minutes to correct the spiritual imbalances in your own family, so that those children and grandchildren coming behind you will not have to experience as much pain in the years to come.

Remember that life is symmetrical and balanced, even in terms of family pain and fear. If you had a difficult relationship with your father, then the mate you attract will have had an equally difficult relationship with his/her mother. If you see the spirit of addiction in your father's family, then you can be sure that the spirit of addiction is also coming from your mother's side of the family. Even if you don't see it, it's there. Often it is hidden a generation or two behind, or it's being manifested as a disease in one generation, but as a visible addiction in another. The pain of life just keeps repeating itself, changing shape until someone steps in to break the cycle.

The spirit of fear and its spawn, addiction, live in your attic and closets until you ask the spirit of love to tell them to leave. It was the violation of spiritual law that created the opportunity for them to occupy your family's house. But a higher spiritual law—the law of Love—gives you the right to throw them out.

Remember, however, that it's not you doing the spiritual work of casting out the spirits of fear and addiction from your house. Your job is to acknowledge their existence and realize you need help from the higher realms. Let go of control and self-judgment. Your own mind has done more than anything else to separate you from receiving love. Put your mind in neutral for a moment. Allow the spirit of love to help you. It does not require perfect faith or perfect comprehension. Just start with a humble heart and a sincere love for your family.

If you have doubts about what you believe, try calling upon the love of Jesus, who is the keeper of the heart. Jesus will not judge your convictions, however misguided they may be. Jesus doesn't care about your religion or which version of the Bible you have read. He doesn't count the number of times you have been naughty or nice. The love of Jesus has never been about merit. It's about grace. Jesus loves your heart, pure and simple. The grace of God flowing through Him is the real instrument that frees your family from the bondage of fear.

Your mission, should you choose to accept it, is to sharpen your focus and clearly indicate which line in your family tree needs the work. It's not enough to stand on your roof, with your arms raised, and shout, "Jesus." The act might bring some cheer to your heart, but it's not likely to free your family from fear and addiction. Shouting from the rooftop is more likely to start a religious war in your neighborhood because well-intended fanaticism usually leads to violence. Quietly focus on your own family for a while. The world can wait for you to be the next messiah.

As you proceed with releasing the fear and addiction from your family, keep in mind that you are not cutting your family off from your life. You are releasing the spirit of the suffering, not the people. You are washing the mud (the fear) off a pot of gold (your family). Keep your family, because it will become the golden pedestal upon which you rise up into heaven.

You may have a special word to describe your act of prayer. You might call it a blessing, a ritual, a ceremony, a clearing, a meditation, or some other name of meaning to you. It doesn't matter.

There are many ways to word your prayer. The following is one example:

"We praise the glory of God, and the grace of His love manifesting through the heart of His son, Jesus. With the aid of this love, we now lovingly release the spirit of all negative emotional control running through our mother's side of the family for four generations, known or unknown to us. This includes the fear of separation and the spirit of addiction. It also includes the spirit of abandonment, the spirit of jealousy, the spirit of anger, and any form of sexual violence. We also release

the spirit of negativity between mother and daughter for four generations, known or unknown to us.

From four generations of our father's side of the family, we lovingly release the spirit of all negative mental control, known or unknown to us. This includes the fear of not receiving love and the spirit of addiction. It also includes the spirit of criticism, the spirits of hate and the loss of recognition. We also release the spirit of sexual violence and the spirit of negativity between father and son, for four generations, known or unknown to us. We lovingly release the combined negativity from both sides of the family for four generations behind us and four generations into the future. We are thankful for the many lessons and gifts we have received as a result of our family's pain. We are also thankful for the divine grace that allows us to be free and to restore the light, peace, and love to our family. We do all of this through the grace of love and the heart of Jesus."

This prayer is only a suggested model. You may add or delete anything you wish. If you have a problem with the name Jesus, you may use 'the vibration of love' in its place. He will not be offended.

Do not expect everything in your life to suddenly turn rosy—quite the contrary. Be prepared for it to feel worse for a short while. Such a prayer for your family has more power than you are aware of, and sadness and suffering will be released. It is rather like standing under an old fruit tree and shaking it so hard that all the dead branches and rotten fruit fall to the ground. Some of the old stuff is likely to fall on your head. It may seem unpleasant, but you have the satisfaction of knowing that only the good remains after all the old debris has been removed. Similarly, destructive spiritual patterns are eliminated, leaving you with a cleaner slate. Do this prayer only when you have the next day off to rest.

Within a day of doing the prayer for your family, it is likely that you or someone in your family will not feel very well. But remember that the pain you experience as a result of the prayer is in the process of being released. It is usually gone within a day but can, sometimes, last for up to three days. Don't try to analyze what's happening or where it is coming from. Instead, head for the bathtub and let the warm water work its magic on you. Allow the pain to be released through the water, rather than through your body.

If you want to make the prayer stronger, write it out by hand first. Then read it aloud three times, and throw the paper into your fireplace. (As demonstrated in the Bible, fire is the last and most powerful form of purification.) Repeat the prayer once a month for four months, adding any new family memories or painful feelings that may arise. Trust yourself and the God who loves you. The prayer is the easy part. The real work is the day-to-day practice of changing the psychological patterns that got your family into trouble in the first place. Changing mental patterns is largely your responsibility. With the aid of a good psychotherapist, it can be made a little easier.

Then comes the task of repairing the physical damage caused by all the years of addiction—the hardest part of all. Rest and a clean diet will work wonders in bringing health, happiness, and prosperity into your life. Building a new life requires time and patience, whereas tearing something down only takes a few minutes. Building something positive is an on-going everyday experience. Prayer can also help in building strength of mind and body in the family. The human mind has a tendency to dwell on the memory of the negative or the fear of something potentially negative in the future. It is important to remember that prayer is also a powerful tool for building positive qualities in yourself and family.

Take the time to realize that you and your family are not the victims of a plot to destroy you. What has happened to your family is the result of ignorance. Without knowledge or conscious awareness, people do things that can have painful consequences for future generations. Families are filled with unconsciousness, which is nothing more than ignorance in action.

Unconsciousness is a killer, but it is also a divinely-inspired mechanism that serves to teach us painful lessons when we violate spiritual laws. Hidden within each painful experience is a gift from God. Every irritation produces a pearl waiting to be discovered. It may be tempting to turn away from the gifts created by family pain and to retreat into denial, but blaming someone else for the problem or just running away from it all is not the answer. In truth, we have played a part in creating every event that has ever happened to us. Through the power of prayer, we also have the opportunity to learn more from our experiences and to reveal the silver lining in the storm cloud.

When something difficult happens to you or your family, take the time to say a prayer of thankfulness to help you surrender to the mystery of the divine. Although we may not understand how or why something painful has come our way, a moment of thankfulness can serve to reveal the gift within the pain.

Remembering to look for the good, and saying a prayer of thankfulness, is particularly appropriate for grandparents, who know a little more about the mysteries of pain. When grandparents say a prayer and look for the deeper meaning of an event, it is remembered by the younger generation. Gradually, the tendency to look for the deeper meaning in life becomes an ever-increasing beacon of light. The inner strength of a grandparent thus becomes a treasure for future generations to enjoy. One of the primary purposes of being a grandparent is to bring freedom.

Ascorbate Protocol

Bowel Tolerance Ascorbate for Maximum Wellness and Control of Acute Infections and Allergic Reactions.

(This information is for educational purposes only and is not intended for use without supervision of a healthcare professional.)

INTRODUCTION:

Ascorbate (Vitamin C) is an important anti-stress substance in the body. When the body is under stress it needs, and will absorb, remarkably large quantities of ascorbate.

The most helpful amount of ascorbate varies greatly from one individual to another and from time to time in the same person. Your body will inform you of the amount of ascorbate it needs by rejecting any excess in the form of diarrhea. You can often improve your energy, immune function, mental clarity, physical comfort, and stress tolerance by taking as much ascorbate as your gut will absorb.

William Blake wrote, "You never know what is enough until you know what is more than enough." You find out about your gut tolerance for ascorbate this way. Your gut tolerance is the maximum amount of ascorbate you can take without getting diarrhea, abdominal discomfort, or excessive gas. The following instructions will enable you to determine how much ascorbate your body needs at any particular time and how to adjust the dose to meet your changing needs.

WARNING!

1. DO NOT begin this protocol without discussing it with a knowledgeable healthcare professional if you have ever had kidney stones._

2. DO NOT continue this protocol for more than two weeks without following the *INSTRUCTIONS FOR LONG TERM USE.*

3. ALWAYS take a high-potency multi-vitamin such as Basic Preventive Five, three capsules or two tablets three times daily while using the bowel tolerance protocol. DO NOT use this protocol without taking this or some similar supplement.

4. A few people do not tolerate large doses of ascorbate. If following this protocol causes abdominal pain, discontinue it.

PROTOCOL FOR MAXIMUM WELLNESS

Use Bronson, Allergy Research Group, AMNI, or Nutricology pure ascorbic acid crystals. These products are available at most healthfood stores and some pharmacies. You can order direct from Bronson by calling 800/235-3200. This is probably your best value—not a small matter if you are taking 15 to 30 grams per day.

Start with 1/4 teaspoonful. This may be placed on the back of the tongue and washed down with water or it may be dissolved in water or in fruit juice if you are not hypersensitive to it. AFTER SWALLOWING THE ASCORBATE, RINSE YOUR MOUTH THOROUGHLY WITH WATER TO REMOVE ASCORBATE FROM YOUR TEETH AND PREVENT ETCHING OF ENAMEL.

Take a dose four times daily, preferably at meals and at bedtime.

Increase each dose by ¼ teaspoon; i.e., ¼ teaspoon, ½ teaspoon, ¾ teaspoon, 1 teaspoon, 1¼ teaspoon, etc. until you develop diarrhea, get abdominal discomfort, or an uncomfortable amount of gas. When any of those things happen, stop taking ascorbate until the symptom subsides, then decrease the dose by ¼ teaspoon per dose until your digestive system is comfortable and you are taking the largest dose compatible with comfort.

At about the time you exceed your bowel tolerance; i.e., develop diarrhea or an excessive amount of gas, you will probably notice an increase in your energy, mental clarity, and sense of well being. Chronic symptoms such as post-nasal drip or joint pain may decrease or stop. So long as you continue to take ascorbate at gut tolerance, you are less likely to get colds and other infections.

Your need for ascorbate will vary with the amount of stress you are under: the more stress, the more ascorbate you need.

Over a period of a month or two, you will probably become quite skillful at estimating the amount of ascorbate that you must take at each dose for maximum benefit without getting diarrhea.

PROTOCOL FOR ACUTE INFECTIONS AND ALLERGIC REACTIONS

Take a dose every hour, increasing by 1/4 teaspoon per dose as described above.

After symptoms are controlled, take your bowel tolerance dose every one to three hours as needed to maintain symptom control. Do *not* stop taking ascorbate after you get diarrhea, but wait until diarrhea stops before taking the next dose. Then, decrease the next dose by ¼ teaspoon. Continue to adjust the dose and the time between doses until you are taking the maximum amount possible with digestive comfort.

INSTRUCTIONS FOR LONG TERM USE. If you take more than 6 grams per day for more than two weeks, wear a Medic-Alert bracelet or necklace and carry a wallet card informing the emergency health care providers about your need for large doses of vitamin C.

INFORMATION FOR MEDICAL CARD

I take vitamin C ____ mg. daily. This has induced enzymes that metabolize vitamin C rapidly. If intake suddenly stops or is drastically reduced, rebound scurvy may result, with risk of shock, hemorrhage, sepsis and wound disruption. To prevent this potentially fatal condition, give me ascorbic acid _____ mg. every 24 hours by mouth or in IV fluids.

RECOMMENDED READING

Learn to use ascorbate more skillfully and effectively by reading:

• Klenner, F.R., Significance of High Daily Intake of Ascorbic Acid in Preventive Medicine

J. of the Int. Acd. of Prev. Med. 1974:45-69.

Dr. Klenner was the pioneer in the use of high dose intravenous ascorbate. He presents fascinating case histories about the power of this treatment in many health problems.

• Cathcart, Robert, Vitamin C, Titrating to Bowel Tolerance, Anascorbemia, and Acute Induced Scurvy

Med. Hypo. 1081; 7: 1359-1376.

Dr. Cathcart has continued Klenner's work and has pioneered the use of oral high dose ascorbate. In this paper, he gives details of how to titrate to bowel tolerance.

• Cathcart, Robert, Vitamin C in the Treatment of Acquired Immune Deficiency Syndrome (AIDS) Med. Hypo. 1984; 14: 423-433

• Cathcart, Robert, Vitamin C treatment of Allergy and the Normally Unprimed State of Antibodies

Med.Hypo. 1986; 21: 307-321.

RESOURCES

Chapter 2

Books by Jonathan V. Wright, M.D. are *Dr. Wright's Guide to Healing with Nutrition, Dr. Wright's Book of Nutritional Therapy, Natural Hormone Replacement,* and *Maximize Your Vitality and Potency for Men Over 40.* All are available at www.tahoma-clinic.com.

Dr. Wright's newsletter is *Nutrition & Healing,* 800/528-0559, Fax 602/943-2363

Chapter 5

Neurofeedback

- A. Martin Wuttke, Institute for Family Wellness, Atlanta, GA, phone 770/395-7526
- EEG Spectrum, national referral center, 818/789-3491
- **Workshops on prayer, meditation, and healing**
- Ron Roth, Celebrating Life Resources, 815/224-3377

Chapter 9

New Franklin Planner: FranklinCovey, 1-800/655-1492, www.franklincovey.com

Chapter 11

The Five Rites of Rejuvenation (video) and *The Eye of Revelation* (book)

- The Blessed Earth Healthfoods, 706/782-6885
- Borderland Sciences Foundation, 707/445-2247

Chapter 12

Adrenal test kits: (Your physician can order)

- Saliva, Diagnos-Techs, 800/878-3787

- Urine, Meridian Valley Clinical Laboratory, 800/234-6825

Chopra Center for Wellness, 800/858-1808

Compounding pharmacists: International Academy of Compounding Pharmacists, 800/927-4227

Flax meal: Phillips Publishing, Inc., 800/705-5559. Ask for priority code #I14012.

Health-related newsletters

- *Health & Healing,* Julian Whitaker, M.D., 800/539-8219
- *Health wisdom for Women,* Christiane Northrup, M.D., 800/211-8561
- *Self Healing,* Andrew Weil, M.D., 800/523-3296

Supplement sources

- AMNI (Advanced Medical Nutrition, Inc.) 800/356-4791
- Bronson Pharmaceutical, 800/235-3200

Water filters: The Sun-Pure Water Filter, Phillips Publishing, Inc., 800/705-5559

Water tests: National Testing Laboratories, Ltd., 800/458-3330

Bibliography

Blake, William, *Selected Poetry and Prose,* New York, Ramdom House, 1953

Bowen, Murray, *Family Therapy in Clinical Practice,* Northvale. NJ, Jason Aronson, 1985

Bucke, Richard M., *Cosmic Consciousness,* New York, E.P. Dutton, 1901

Byrom, Thomas, *Dhammapada, The, the Sayings of Buddha,* New York, Vintage Books, 1979

Campbell, Don, ed., *Music Physician for Time to Come,* Wheaton, IL, Theosophical Publishing House

Chopra, Deepak, *Creating Affluence,* San Rafael, CA, New Work Library, 1993

_____, *Perfect Health,* New York, Harmony Books, 1991

_____, *Quantum Healing,* New York, Bantum, 1989

_____, *Sacred Verses, Healing Sounds,* San Rafael, CA, New World Library, 1994

_____, *Seven Spiritual Laws of Success, The,* San Rafael, CA, New World Library, 1994

_____, *Ageless Body, Timeless Mind,* New York, Harmony Books, 1993

Covey, Stephen, *7 Habits of Highly Effective People, The,* New York, Fireside Books, 1989

Dyer, Wayne W., *Real Magic,* New York, Harper Collins, 1989

Dylan, Bob, *Writings and Drawings by Bob Dylan,* New York, Alfred A. Knorf, 1973

Frankl, Viktor E., *Man's Search for Meaning,* Boston, MA, Beacon Press, 1959

Gibran, Kahlil, *Prophet, The,* New York, Alfred A Knorf, 1923

Kapleau, Phillip, *Three Pillars of Zen,* The, New York, John Weatherhill, Inc., 1967

_____, *Wheel of Death, The,* London, George Allen & Unwin, Ltd., 1972

_____, *Wheel of Life and Death,* The, New York, Doubleday, 1989

Lanier, Sydney, *Poems of Sidney Lanier,* Athens, GA, University of Georgia Press, 1967

Myss, Caroline, *Anatomy of the Spirit,* New York, Three Rivers Press, 1996

_____, *Energy Anatomy,* Boulder, CO, Sounds True, 1996

_____, *Why People Don't Heal and How They Can,* New York, Harmony Books, 1997

Redfield, James, *Tenth Insight,* The, New York, Warner Books, 1996

_____, *Celestine Vision,* The, New York, Warner Books, 1997

_____, *Celestine Prophecy,* The, An Experiential Guide, New York, Warner Books, 1997

Roth, Ron, *Healing Path of Prayer, The,* New York, Harmony books, 1997

Sears, Barry, *Zone, The,* New York, Harper Collins, 1995

Tagore, Rabindranath, *Gitanjali,* New York, Macmillan Publishing Company, 1971

Thoreau, Henry D., *Walden,* New York, Random House, 1950

Habits are at first cobwebs, then cables.

—Spanish Proverb

THE WHOLE SELF

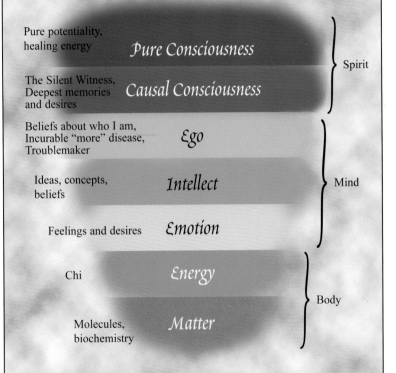

Pure potentiality, healing energy — *Pure Consciousness*

The Silent Witness, Deepest memories and desires — *Causal Consciousness*

} Spirit

Beliefs about who I am, Incurable "more" disease, Troublemaker — *Ego*

Ideas, concepts, beliefs — *Intellect*

Feelings and desires — *Emotion*

} Mind

Chi — *Energy*

Molecules, biochemistry — *Matter*

} Body

Index

Order Form

Fax orders: (706) 782-1532

Telephone orders: 1-800-834-4167.
Have your MasterCard or VISA ready.

Postal orders: Healthspirit Press, Jack Woodard, P.O. Box 8064, Clayton, GA 30525-0806, USA • Tel: (706) 782-1219

Please send ____ copies of *Healthspan: Claim Your Birthright to Holistic Health and Happiness from Here to 100.*

I understand that I may return these books for a full refund—for any reason, no questions asked.

___ Please add my name to your mailing list. I understand that you do not make your mailing list available to any other organization or individual.

Company name: _____

Name: _____

Address: _____

City: _____State: _____ Zip: _____-_____

Telephone:_____Fax:_____

E-mail address_____

Sales tax: Please add 7% for books shipped to Georgia addresses.
Shipping: $4.00 for first book and $2.00 for each additional book

Payment: Cheque ___, MasterCard ___, VISA ___

Card number: _____

Exp. Date: ___/___

Name on card: _____